BOTH GIRLS AND BOYS, MEN AND WOMEN, CAN EXCEL IN VARIOUS AREAS, AND IT'S IMPORTANT TO CELEBRATE AND SUPPORT EACH PERSON'S UNIQUE ABILITIES AND POTENTIAL.

THESE FIELDS ARE NOT EXCLUSIVE TO ANY GENDER, AND INDIVIDUAL SUCCESS IS DETERMINED BY SKILLS, PASSION, AND DEDICATION RATHER THAN GENDER. WOMEN HAVE MADE SIGNIFICANT CONTRIBUTIONS IN VARIOUS DOMAINS DUE TO THEIR COMMITMENT, TALENT, AND OPPORTUNITIES AVAILABLE TO THEM. IT'S IMPORTANT TO RECOGNIZE AND CELEBRATE THESE ACHIEVEMENTS WITHOUT MAKING GENERALIZATIONS ABOUT GENDER SUPERIORITY.

IT IS IMPORTANT TO AVOID MAKING BROAD GENERALIZATIONS ABOUT WHAT ONE GENDER IS BETTER AT THAN THE OTHER, AS ABILITIES AND STRENGTHS VARY WIDELY AMONG INDIVIDUALS REGARDLESS OF THEIR GENDER.

IT'S ESSENTIAL TO EMPHASIZE THAT GENDER SHOULD NOT BE A BASIS FOR COMPARISON OR SUPERIORITY. BOTH GIRLS AND BOYS, MEN AND WOMEN, HAVE THEIR OWN UNIQUE QUALITIES AND STRENGTHS. RATHER THAN FOCUSING ON DIFFERENCES, IT'S MORE PRODUCTIVE TO PROMOTE EQUALITY AND RECOGNIZE THE VALUE OF EVERY INDIVIDUAL REGARDLESS OF THEIR GENDER.

IT'S ESSENTIAL TO RECOGNIZE THAT THESE ARE GENERAL TRENDS, AND INDIVIDUAL HEALTH OUTCOMES CAN VARY WIDELY. BOTH GENDERS HAVE UNIQUE HEALTH CHALLENGES AND STRENGTHS.

100 reasons why girls are better than boys

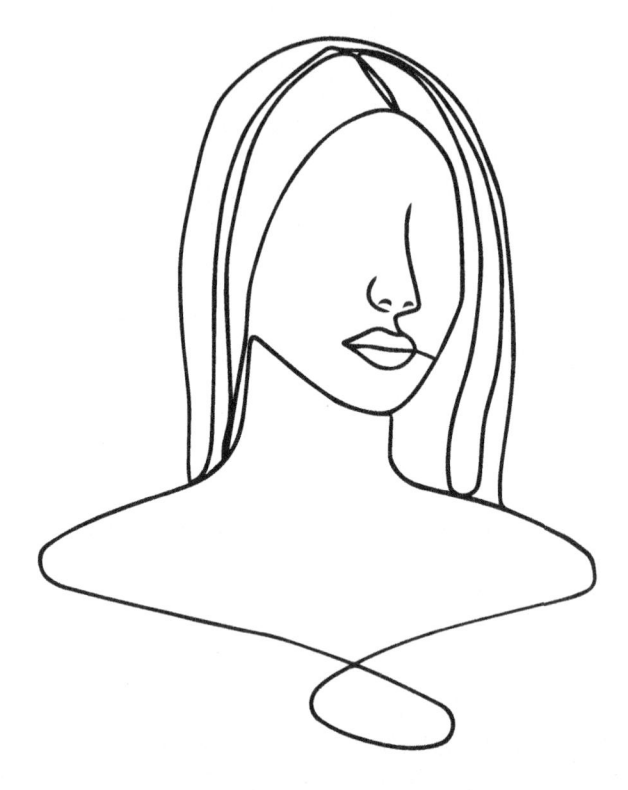

LONGEVITY: ON AVERAGE, WOMEN TEND TO LIVE LONGER THAN MEN IN MANY COUNTRIES.

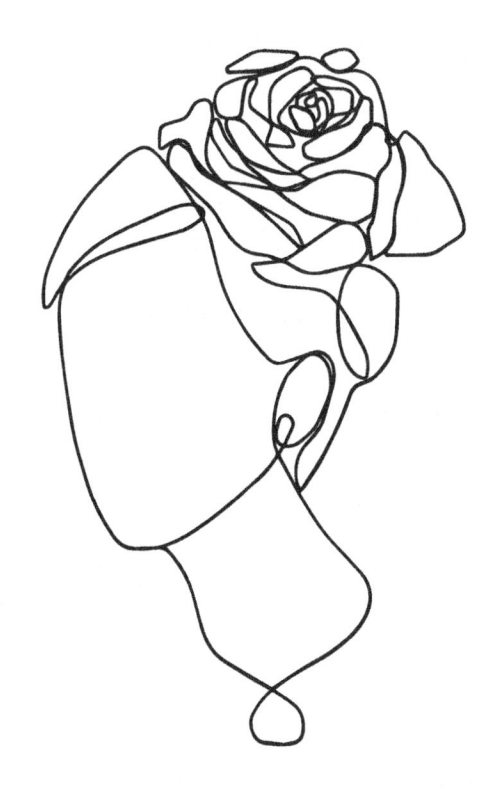

STRONGER IMMUNE RESPONSE: SOME STUDIES SUGGEST THAT FEMALES GENERALLY EXHIBIT STRONGER IMMUNE RESPONSES TO INFECTIONS AND VACCINATIONS.

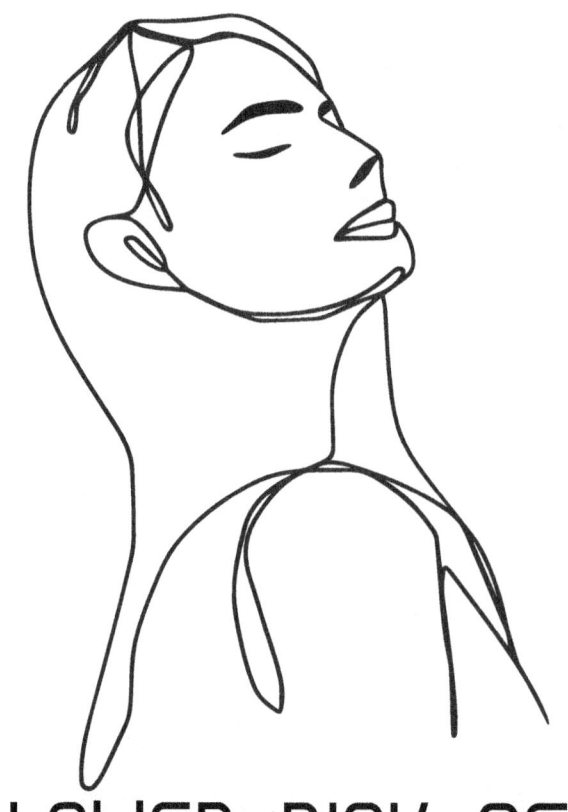

LOWER RISK OF CARDIOVASCULAR DISEASE: PRE-MENOPAUSAL WOMEN OFTEN HAVE A LOWER RISK OF HEART DISEASE COMPARED TO MEN OF THE SAME AGE.

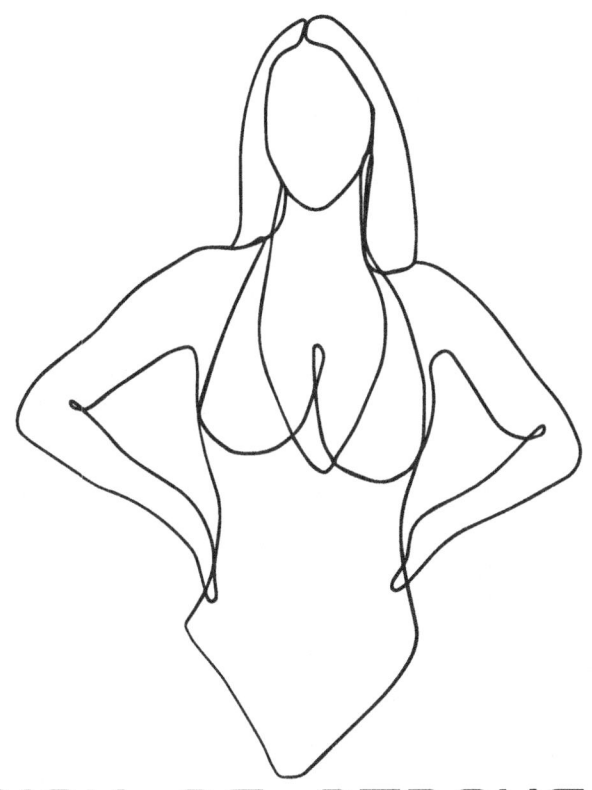

LOWER RISK OF STROKE: WOMEN TEND TO HAVE A LOWER RISK OF STROKE, ESPECIALLY AT A YOUNGER AGE.

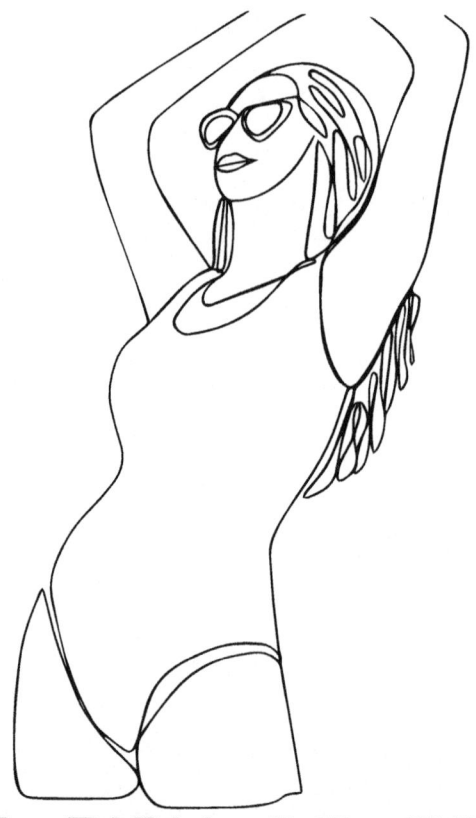

LOWER RISK OF CERTAIN CANCERS: RATES OF CERTAIN TYPES OF CANCERS, SUCH AS LUNG AND COLORECTAL CANCER, TEND TO BE LOWER IN WOMEN.

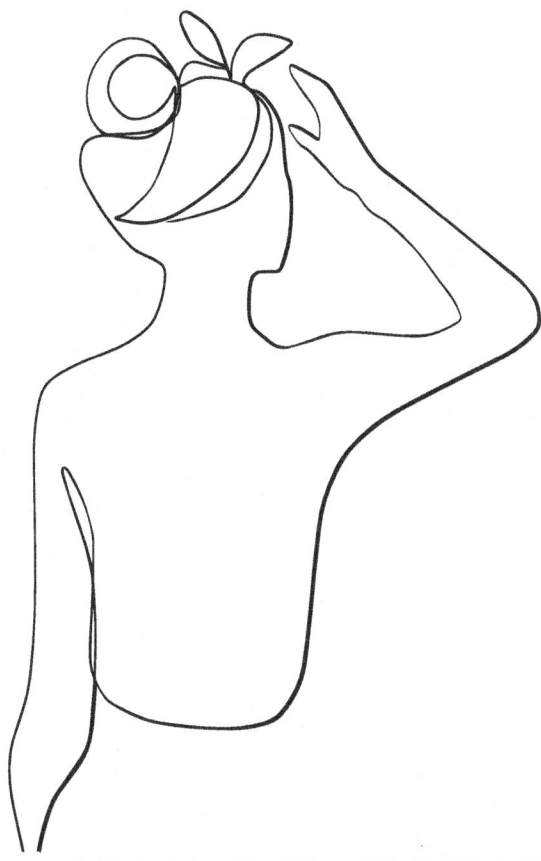

LOWER RISK OF PARKINSON'S DISEASE: PARKINSON'S DISEASE IS MORE COMMON IN MEN THAN WOMEN.

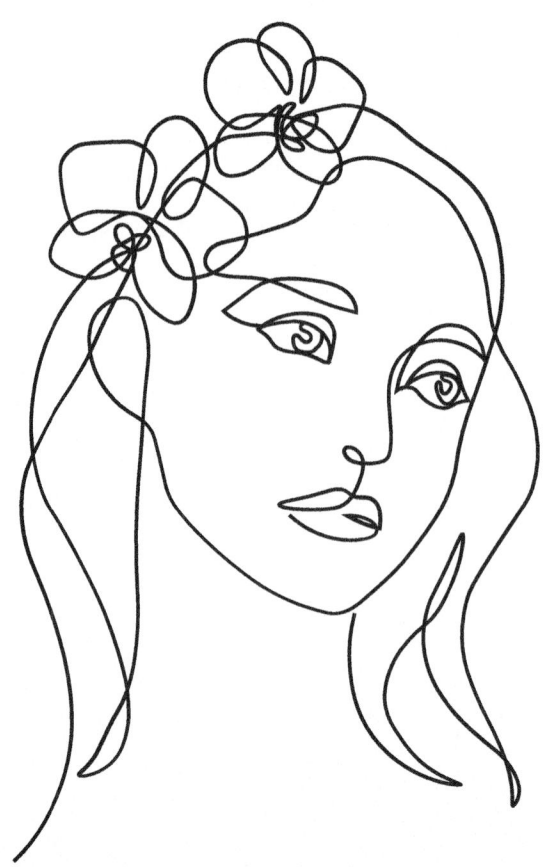

BETTER PAIN TOLERANCE: SOME STUDIES SUGGEST THAT WOMEN MAY HAVE A HIGHER PAIN TOLERANCE.

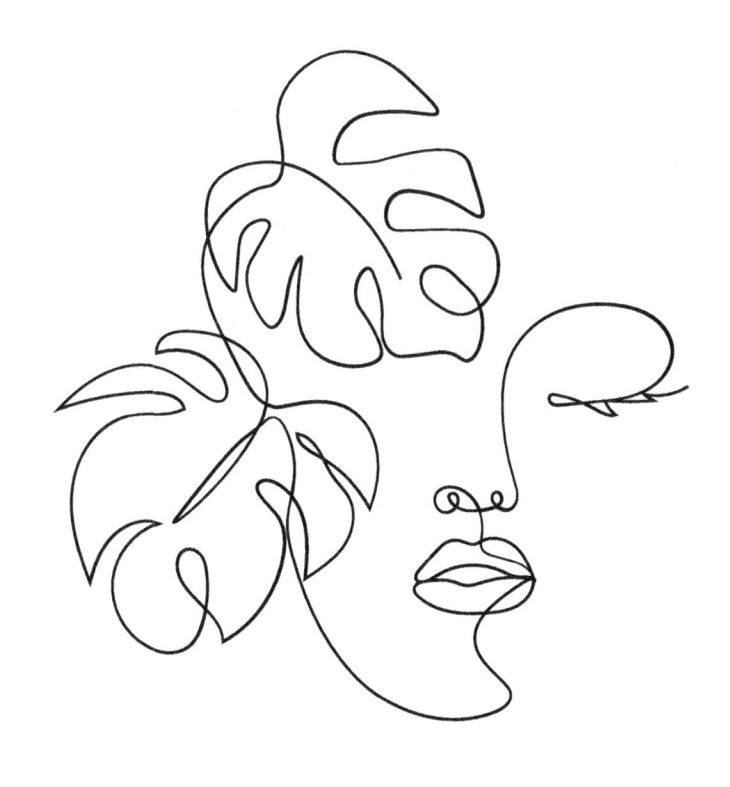

LOWER RISK OF AUTISM SPECTRUM DISORDERS: BOYS ARE MORE LIKELY TO BE DIAGNOSED WITH AUTISM SPECTRUM DISORDERS.

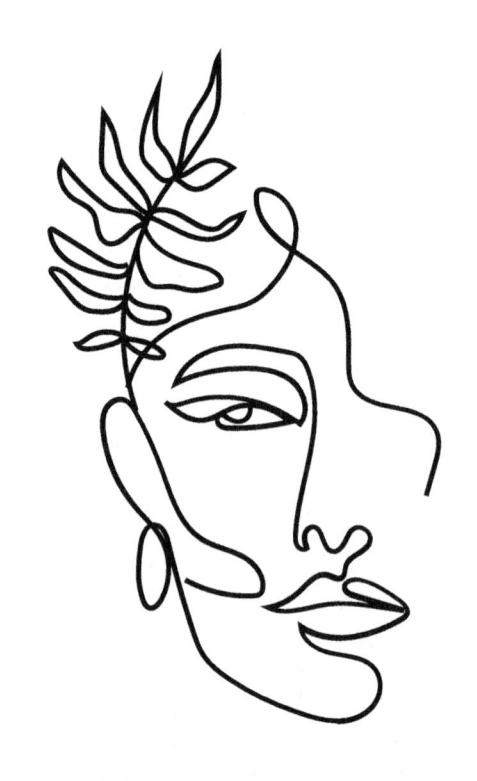

HIGHER LIFE SATISFACTION: RESEARCH HAS SHOWN THAT WOMEN OFTEN REPORT HIGHER LEVELS OF LIFE SATISFACTION.

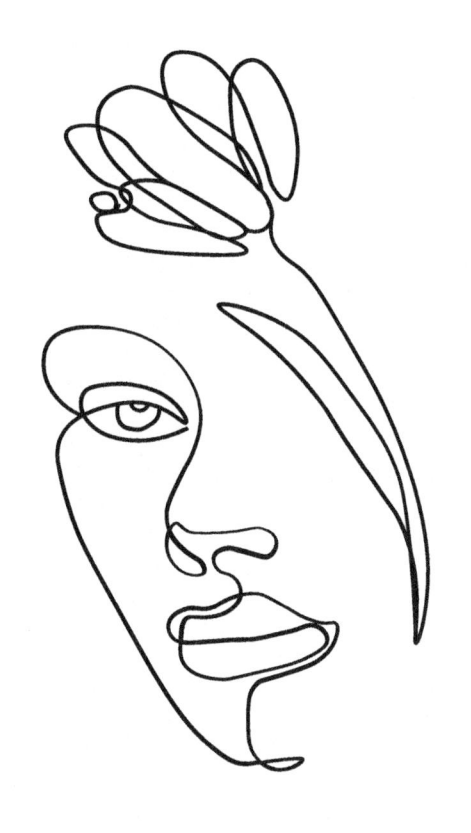

BETTER MENTAL HEALTH HELP-SEEKING: WOMEN ARE OFTEN MORE LIKELY TO SEEK HELP FOR MENTAL HEALTH ISSUES.

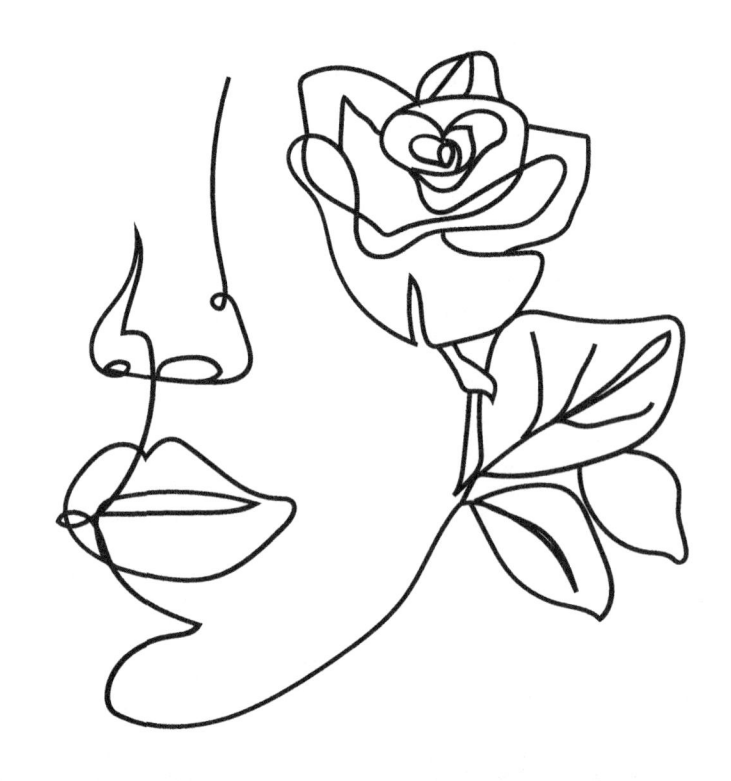

LOWER RISK OF OCCUPATIONAL HAZARDS: WOMEN MAY BE EXPOSED TO FEWER OCCUPATIONAL HAZARDS.

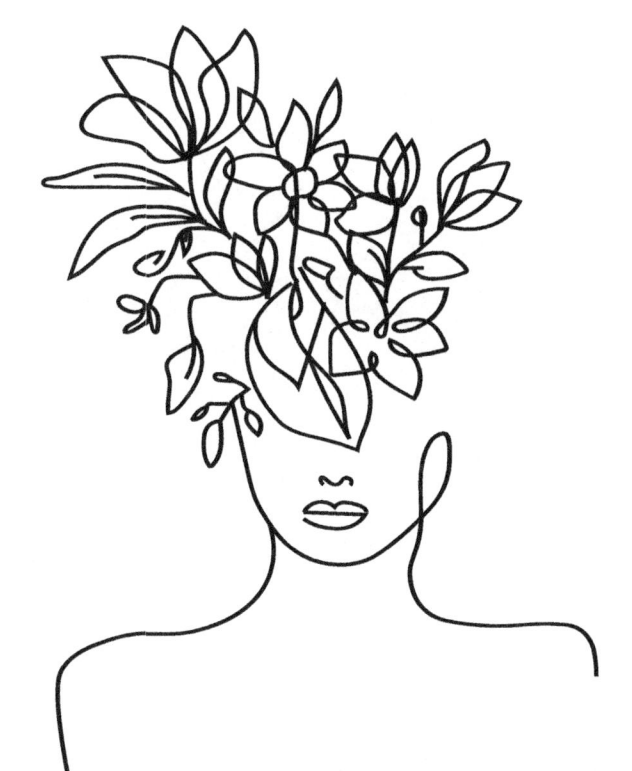

HEALTHIER EATING HABITS: WOMEN MAY BE MORE CONSCIOUS OF THEIR DIETS AND HAVE HEALTHIER EATING HABITS.

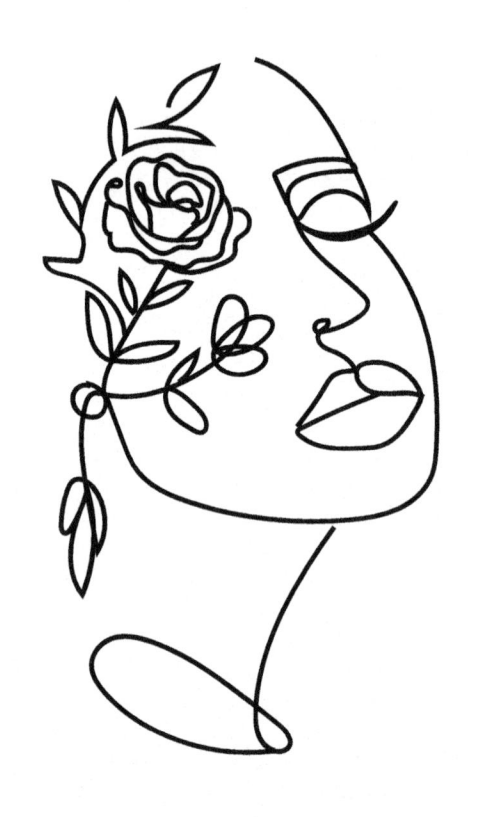

LOWER RISK OF SUBSTANCE ABUSE: WOMEN TEND TO HAVE LOWER RATES OF SUBSTANCE ABUSE COMPARED TO MEN.

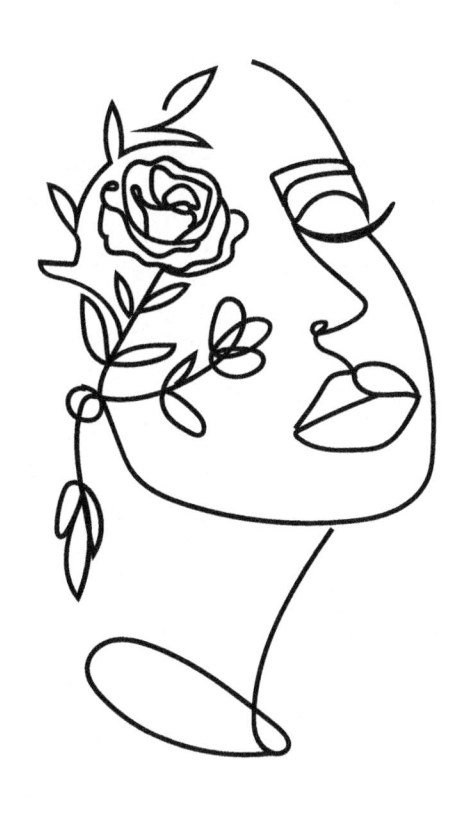

LOWER RISK OF HEAD INJURIES: MEN ARE MORE LIKELY TO EXPERIENCE HEAD INJURIES.

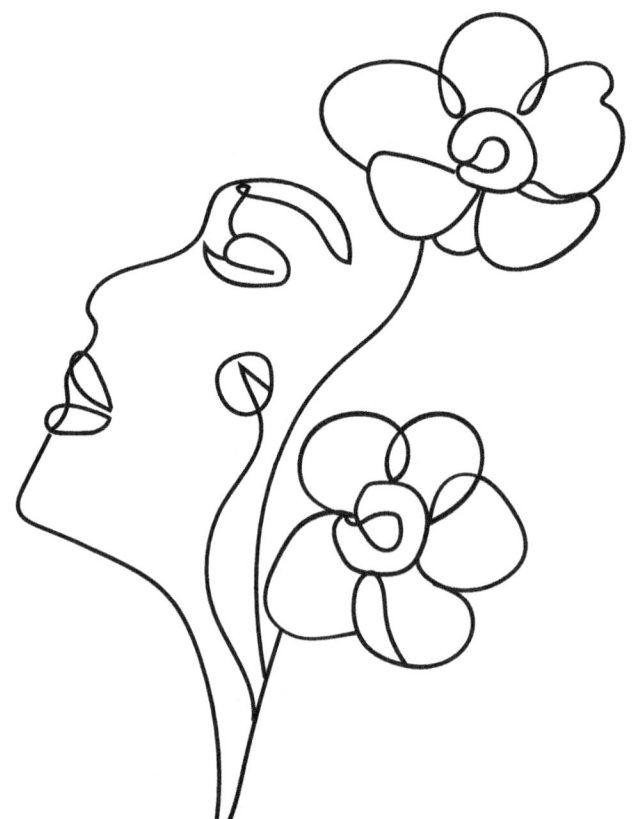

LESS RISKY BEHAVIORS: YOUNG MEN ARE MORE LIKELY TO ENGAGE IN RISKY BEHAVIORS.

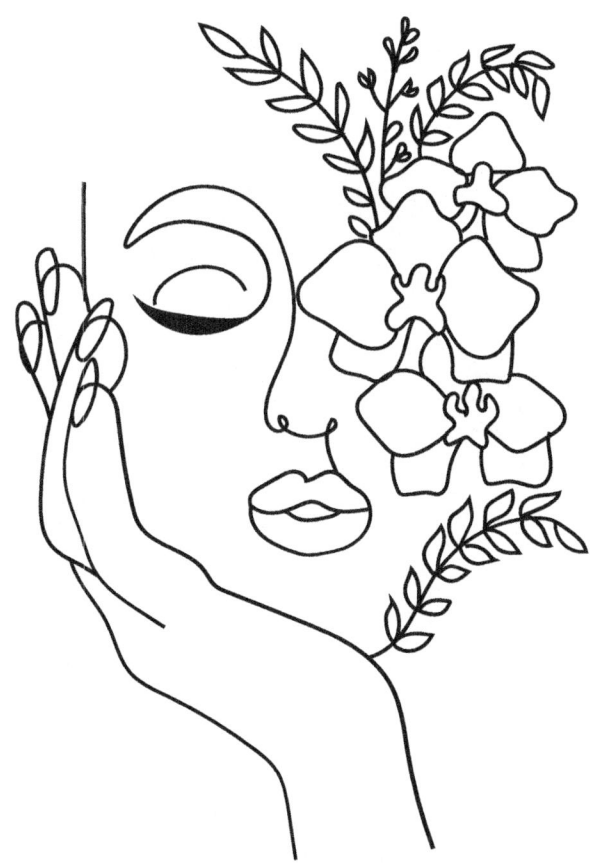

HORMONAL DIFFERENCES: HORMONAL DIFFERENCES BETWEEN GENDERS MAY CONTRIBUTE TO HEALTH ADVANTAGES.

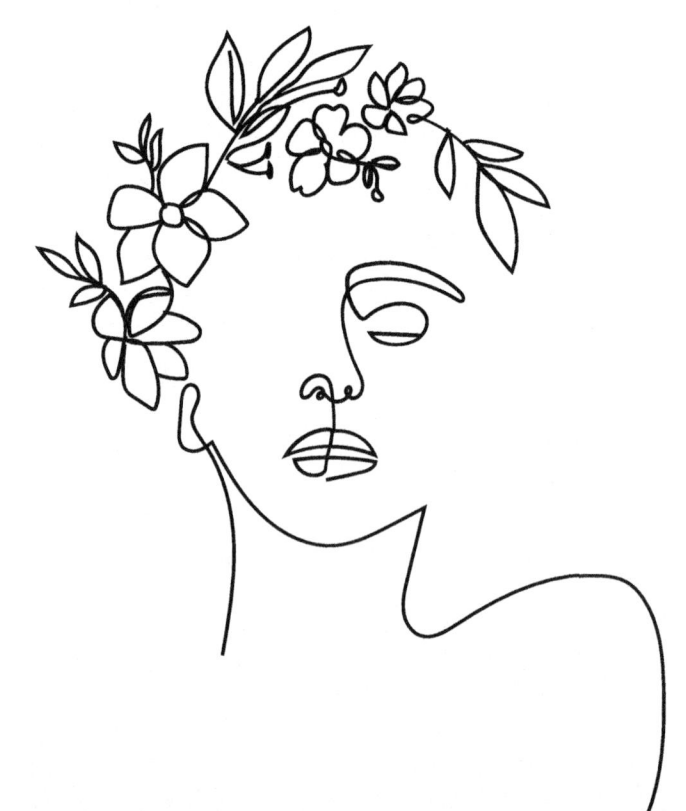

STRONGER SOCIAL SUPPORT NETWORKS: WOMEN OFTEN EXCEL IN BUILDING AND MAINTAINING SOCIAL SUPPORT NETWORKS, WHICH CAN POSITIVELY IMPACT MENTAL AND EMOTIONAL WELL-BEING.

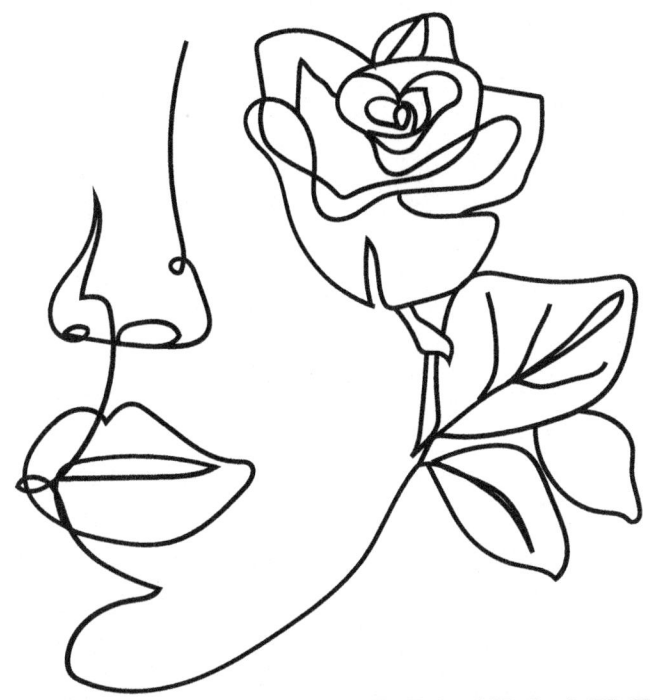

LOWER RISK OF COMPLICATIONS FROM INFECTIONS: WOMEN MAY HAVE A LOWER RISK OF COMPLICATIONS FROM CERTAIN INFECTIONS.

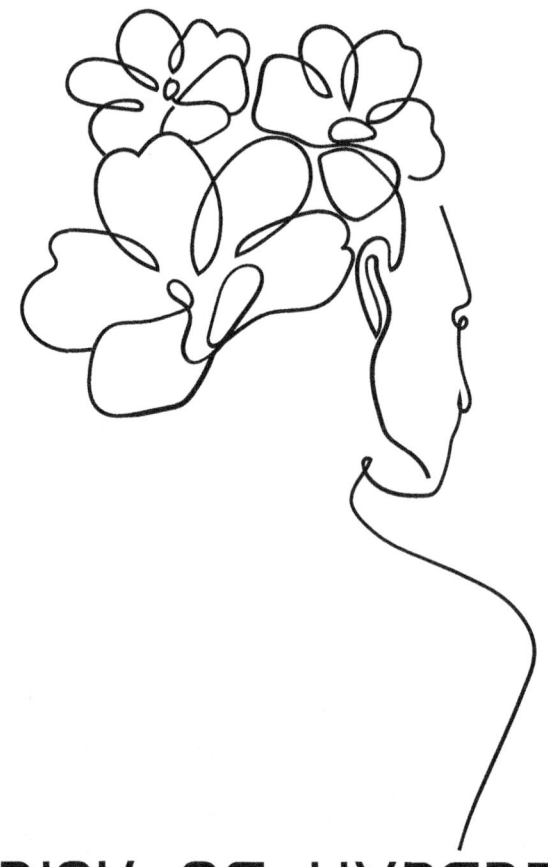

LOWER RISK OF HYPERTENSION: HYPERTENSION (HIGH BLOOD PRESSURE) IS LESS COMMON IN WOMEN BEFORE MENOPAUSE.

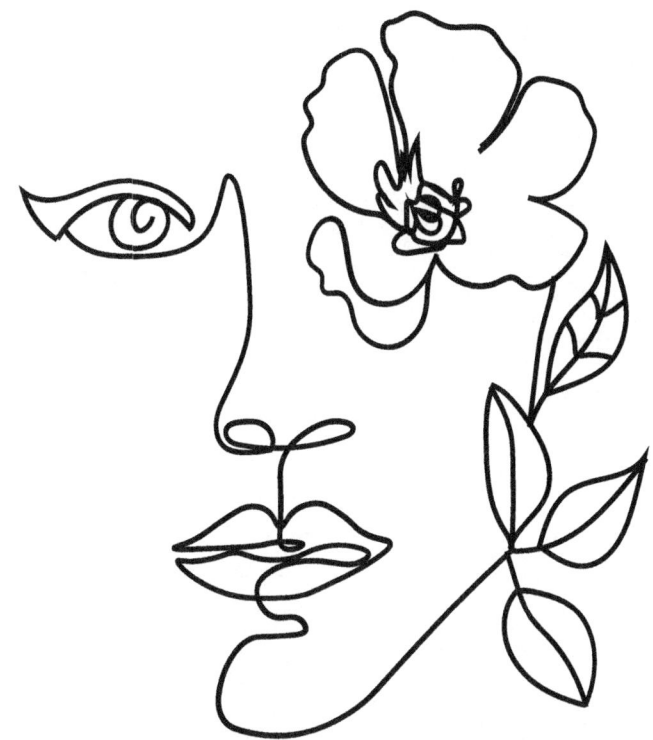

HEALTHIER AGING: WOMEN MAY EXPERIENCE A SLOWER RATE OF PHYSICAL DECLINE IN OLDER AGE.

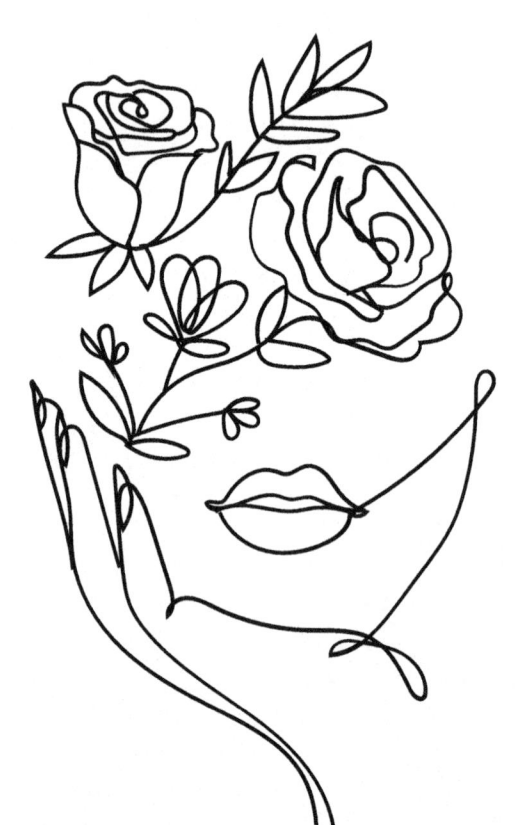

BETTER BONE HEALTH: WOMEN TYPICALLY HAVE HIGHER BONE DENSITY, WHICH CAN CONTRIBUTE TO BETTER BONE HEALTH.

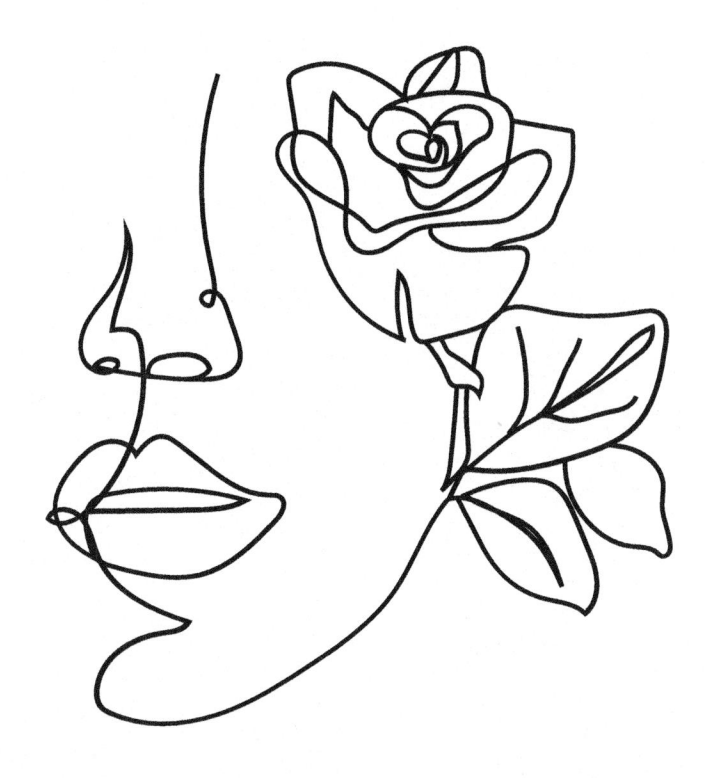

LESS RISKY DRIVING HABITS: MEN ARE MORE LIKELY TO ENGAGE IN RISKY DRIVING BEHAVIORS.

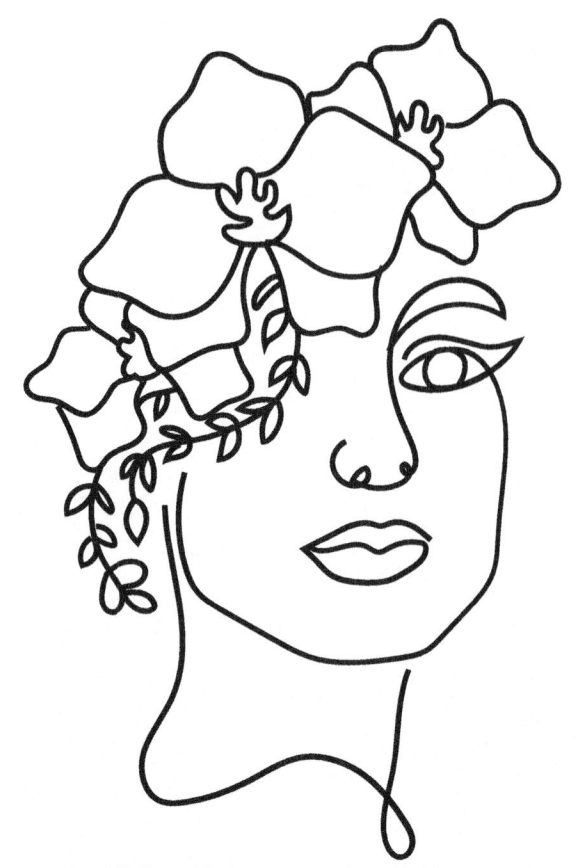

HIGHER HEALTH LITERACY: WOMEN MAY HAVE HIGHER HEALTH LITERACY AND AWARENESS.

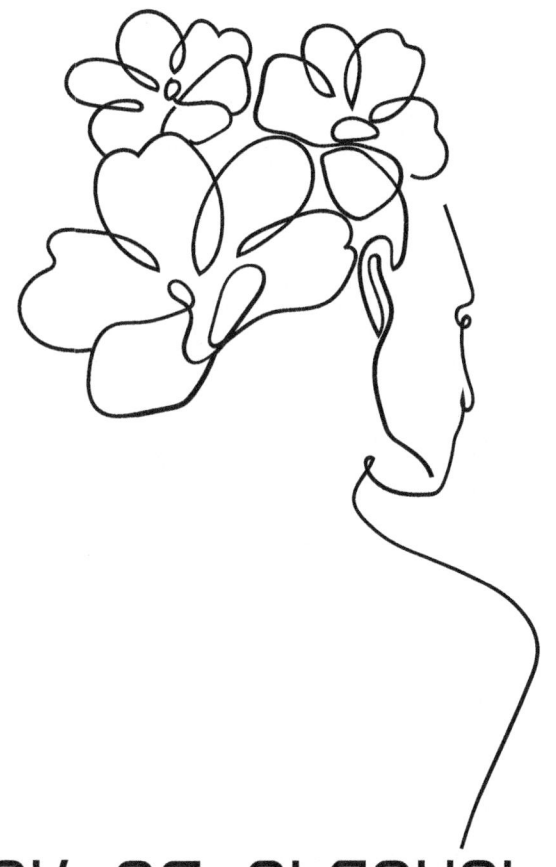

LOWER RISK OF ALCOHOL-RELATED ISSUES: MEN ARE MORE LIKELY TO EXPERIENCE ALCOHOL-RELATED PROBLEMS.

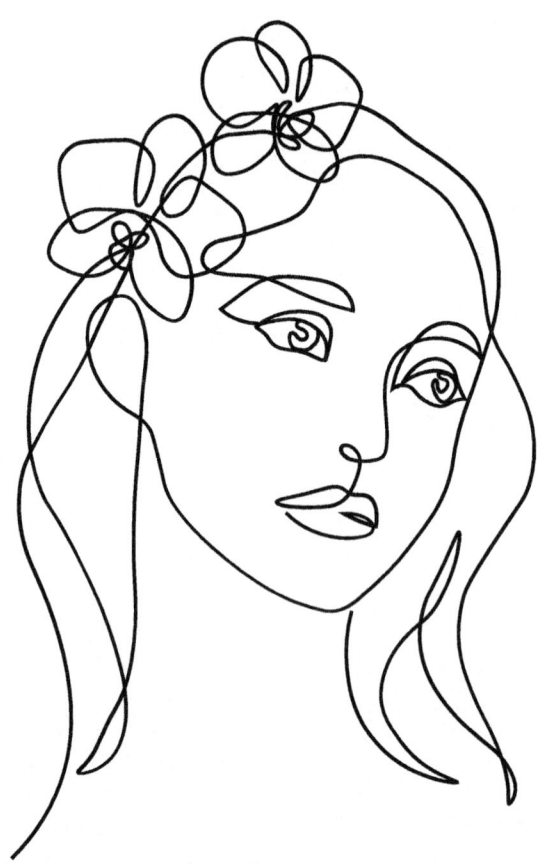

BETTER SLEEP PATTERNS: WOMEN OFTEN REPORT BETTER SLEEP QUALITY.

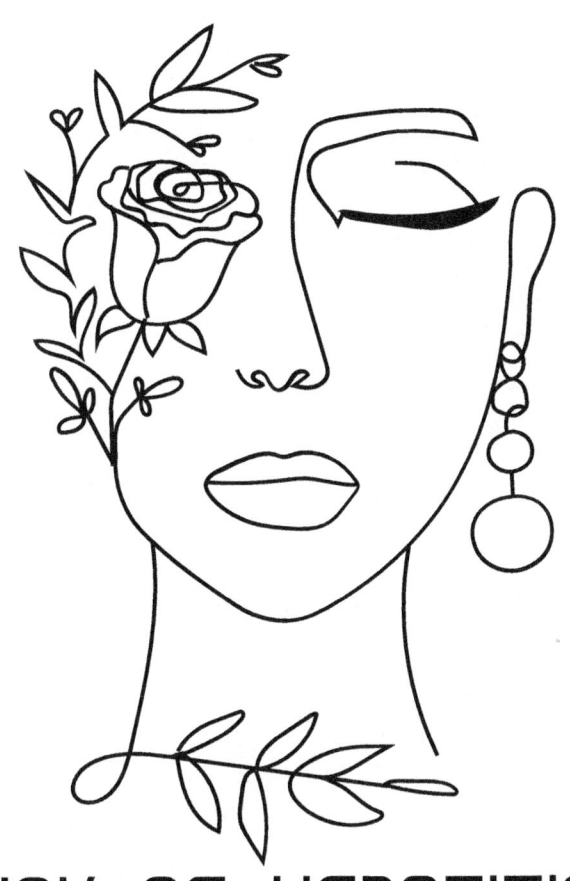

LOWER RISK OF HEPATITIS C: MEN ARE MORE LIKELY TO BE INFECTED WITH HEPATITIS C.

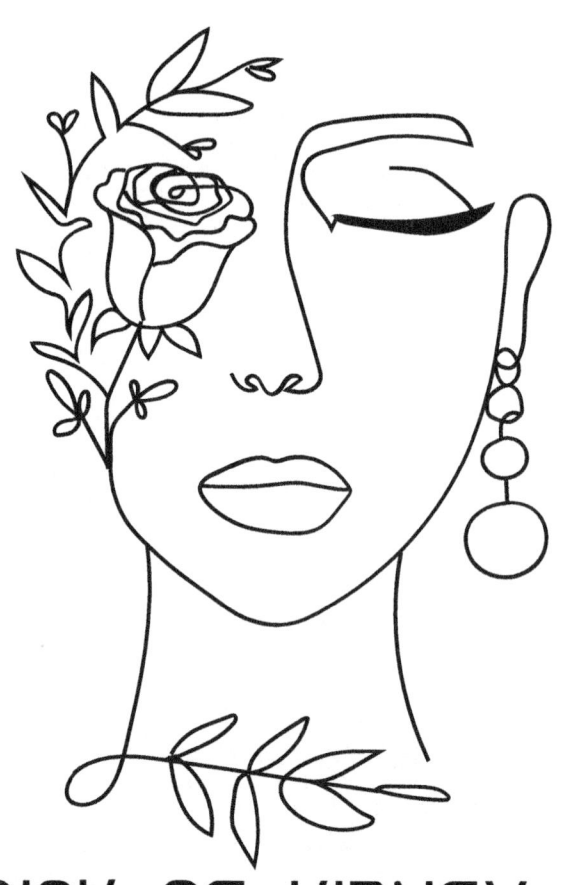

LOWER RISK OF KIDNEY STONES:
KIDNEY STONES ARE MORE
COMMON IN MEN.

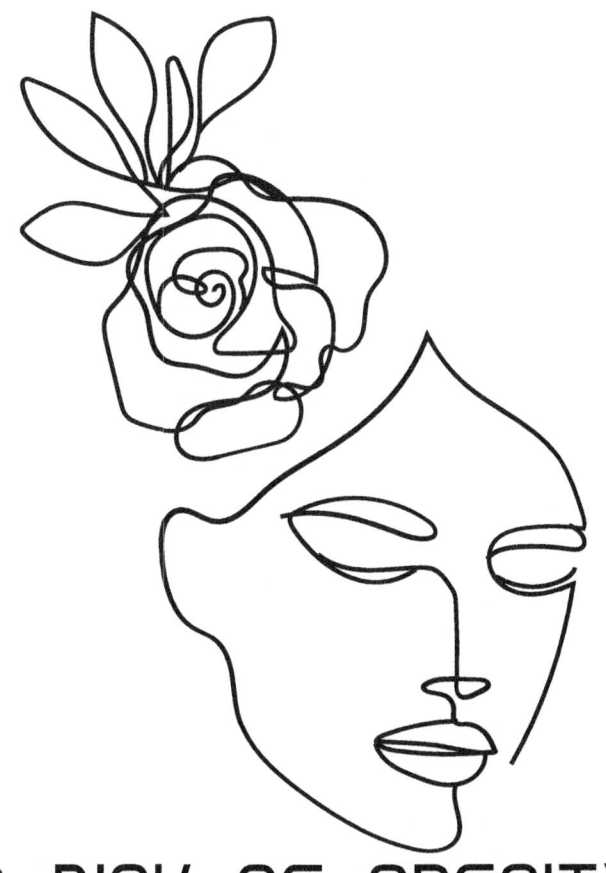

LOWER RISK OF OBESITY: WOMEN MAY HAVE A LOWER RISK OF OBESITY, ESPECIALLY IN CERTAIN AGE GROUPS.

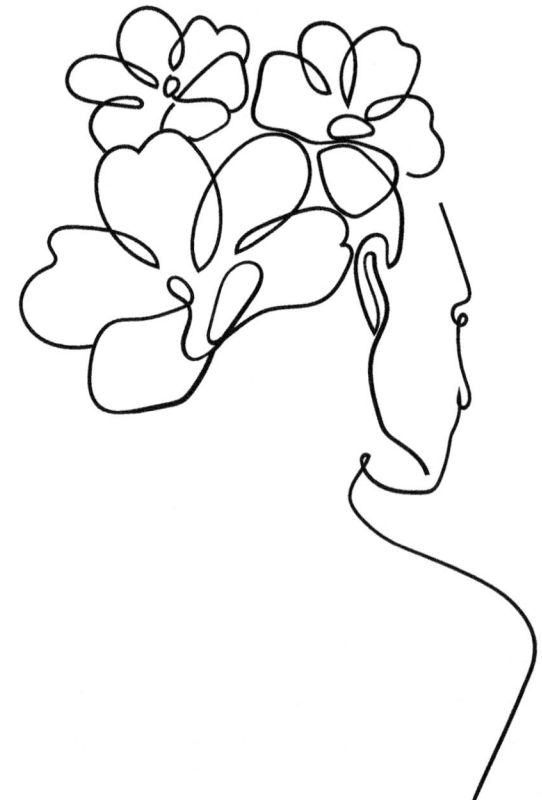

BETTER STRESS MANAGEMENT: WOMEN MAY HAVE BETTER STRESS-COPING MECHANISMS.

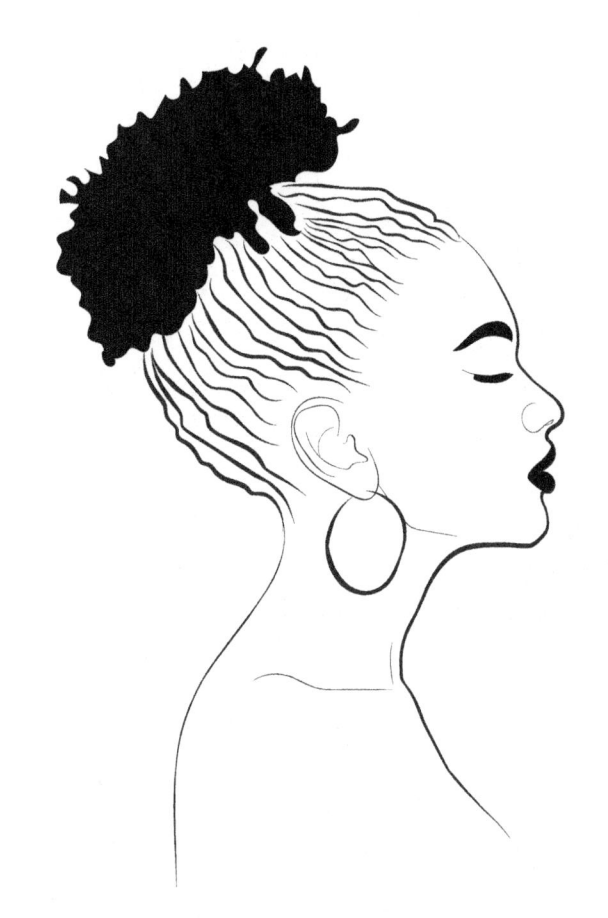

GIRLS MAY BE MORE ENCOURAGED TO EXPRESS THEIR EMOTIONS OPENLY AND DISCUSS THEIR FEELINGS WITH OTHERS.

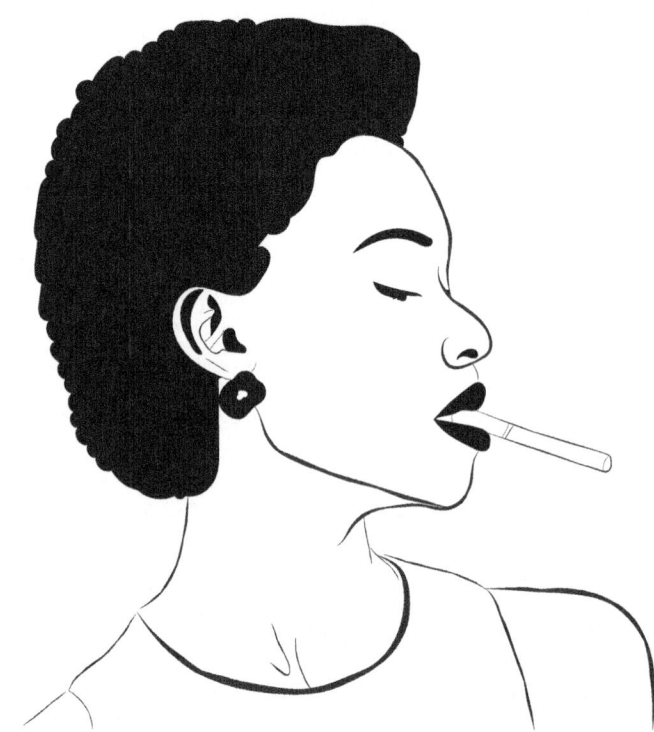

GIRLS ARE OFTEN PRAISED FOR THEIR STRONG COMMUNICATION SKILLS AND MAY ENGAGE IN MORE CONVERSATION AND SOCIAL INTERACTION.

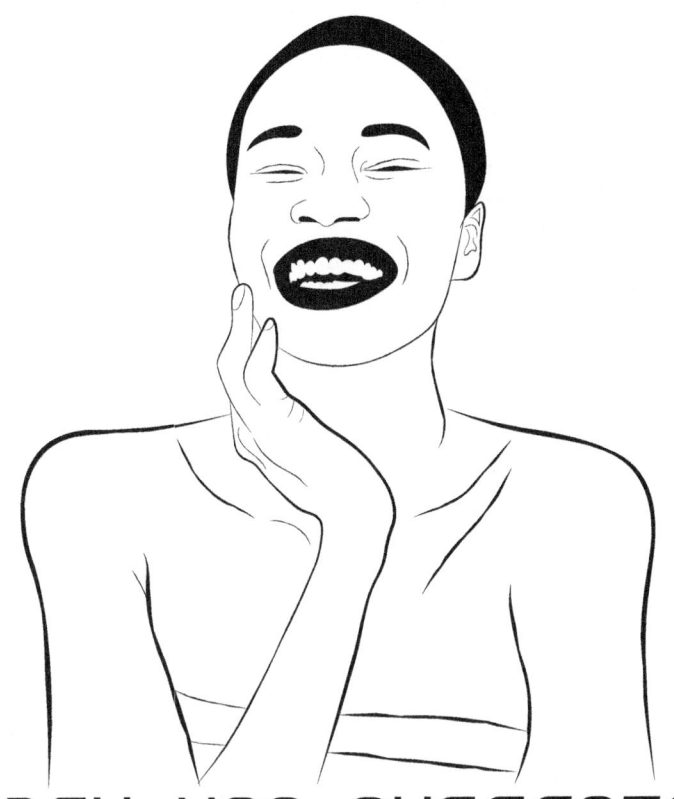

RESEARCH HAS SUGGESTED THAT GIRLS MAY DISPLAY HIGHER LEVELS OF EMPATHY, WHICH CAN CONTRIBUTE TO THEIR SOCIAL INTERACTIONS.

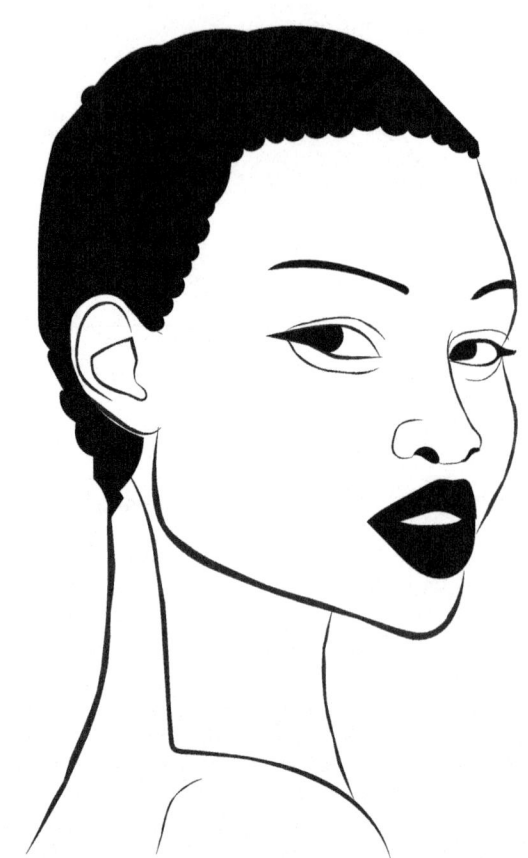

GIRLS MAY PLACE A STRONG EMPHASIS ON THE QUALITY AND DEPTH OF THEIR FRIENDSHIPS.

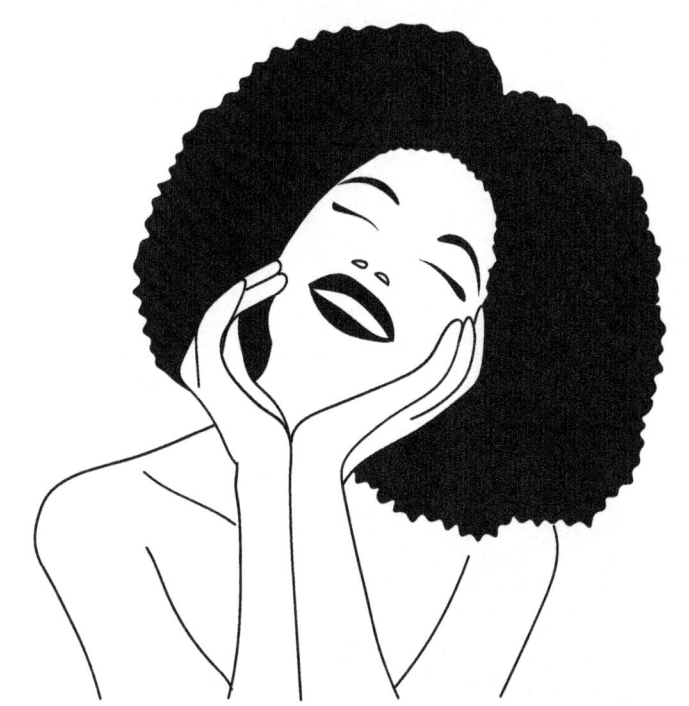

GIRLS MIGHT BE MORE INCLINED TO ENGAGE IN COOPERATIVE AND COLLABORATIVE ACTIVITIES.

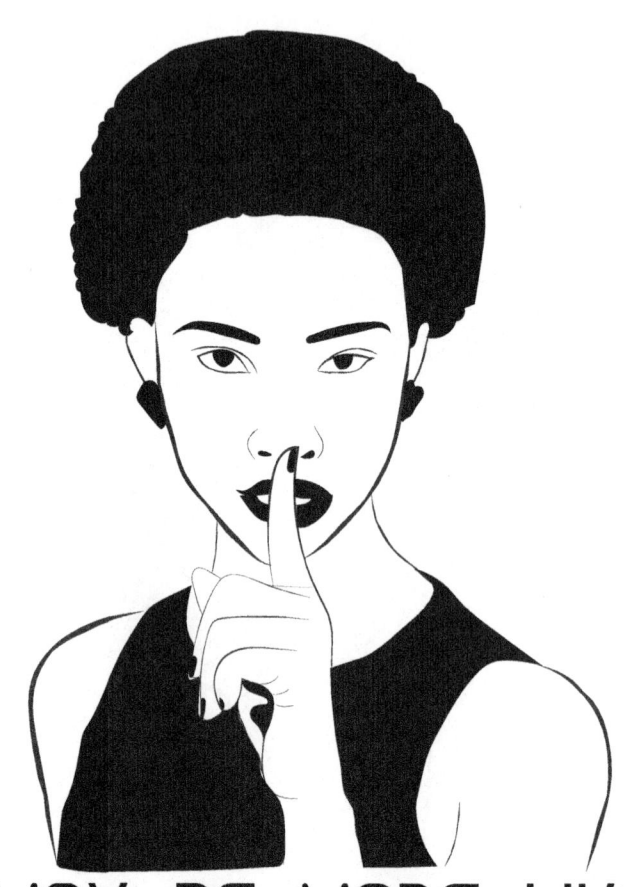

GIRLS MAY BE MORE LIKELY TO SHARE PERSONAL EXPERIENCES AND SEEK SUPPORT FROM FRIENDS.

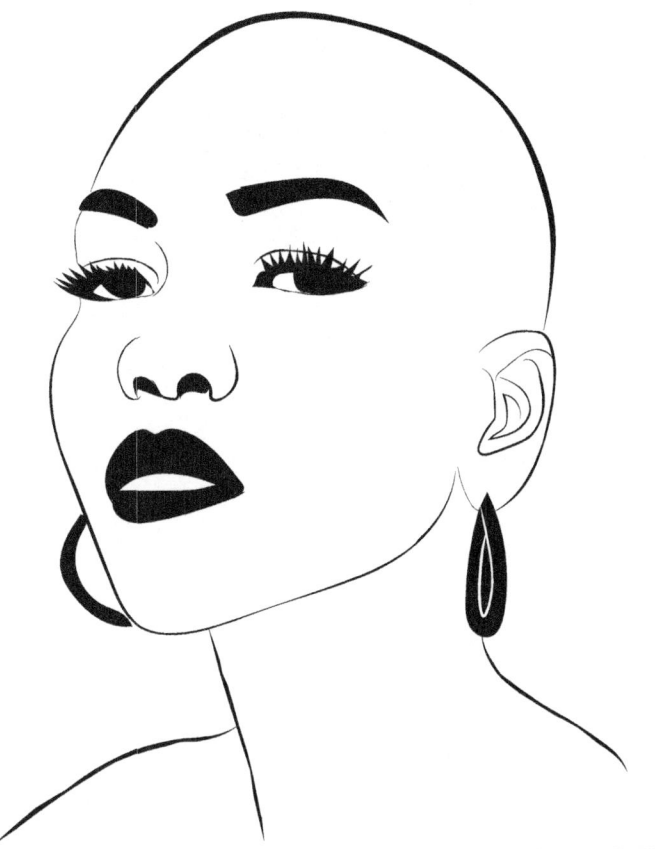

GIRLS MAY ENJOY PARTICIPATING IN GROUP ACTIVITIES AND GATHERINGS.

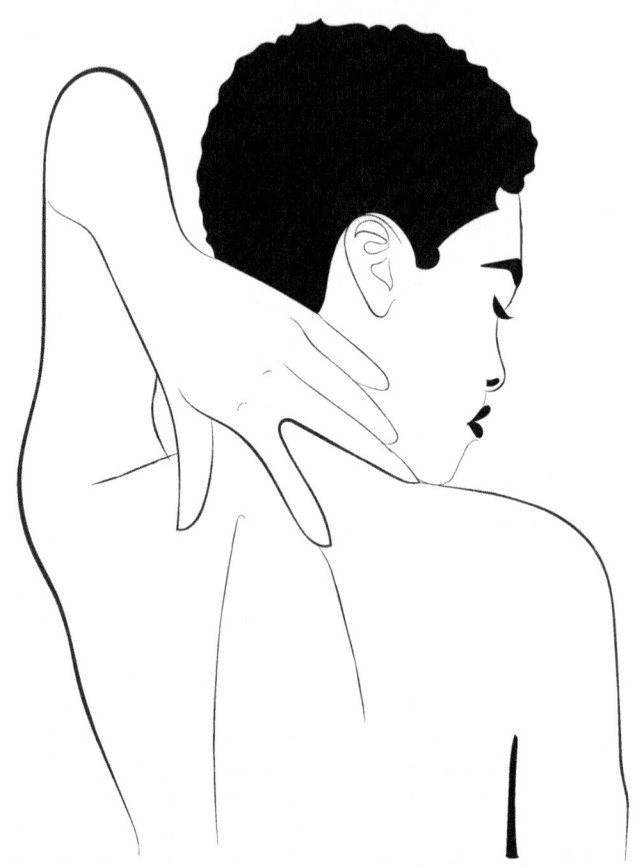

SOME RESEARCH SUGGESTS THAT GIRLS MAY USE MORE COLLABORATIVE AND LESS CONFRONTATIONAL CONFLICT RESOLUTION STRATEGIES.

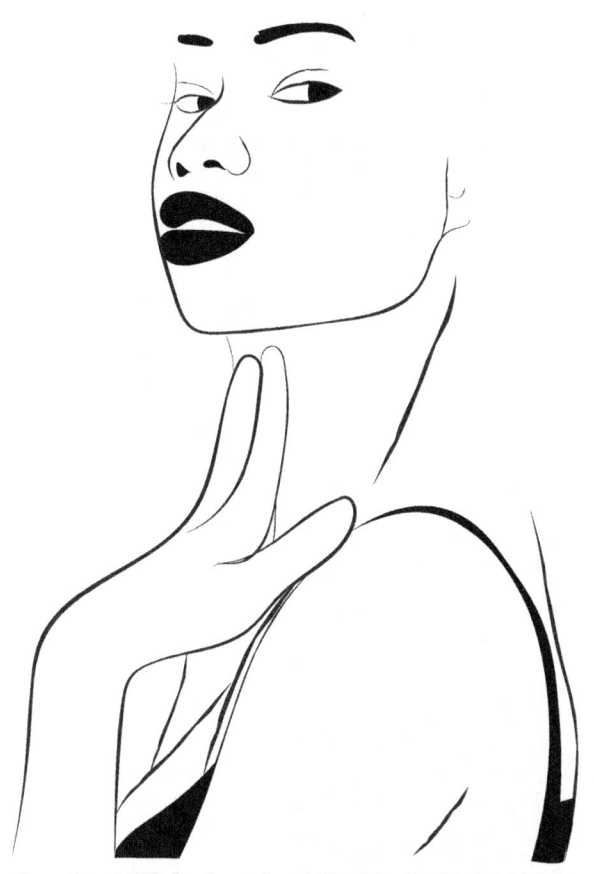

WOMEN MAY MAINTAIN LARGER AND MORE INTERCONNECTED SOCIAL NETWORKS.

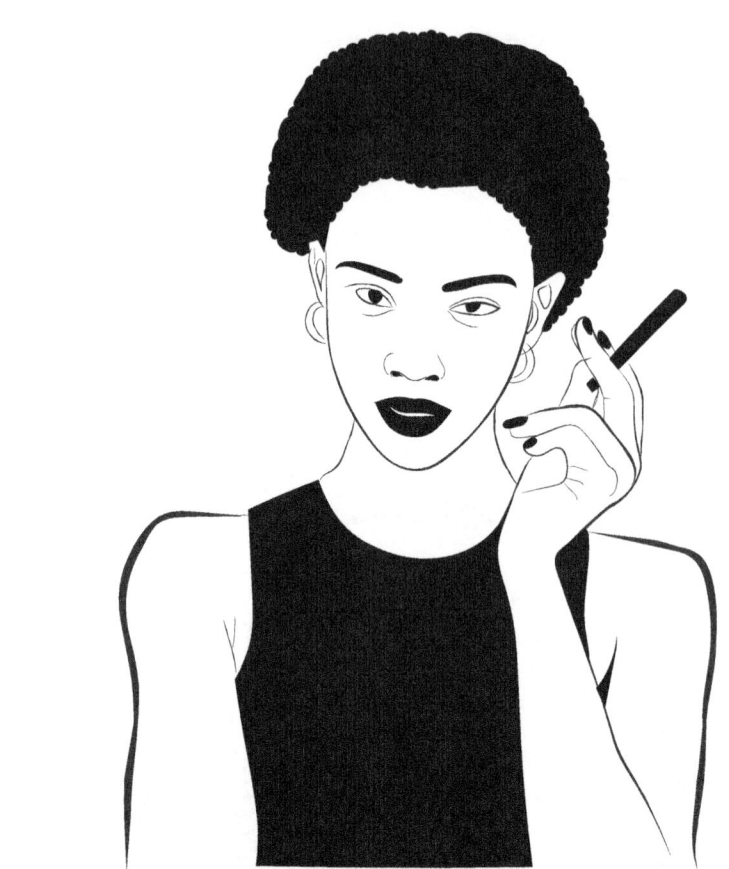

MENTAL HEALTH COUNSELING:
MANY MENTAL HEALTH
PROFESSIONALS ARE WOMEN.

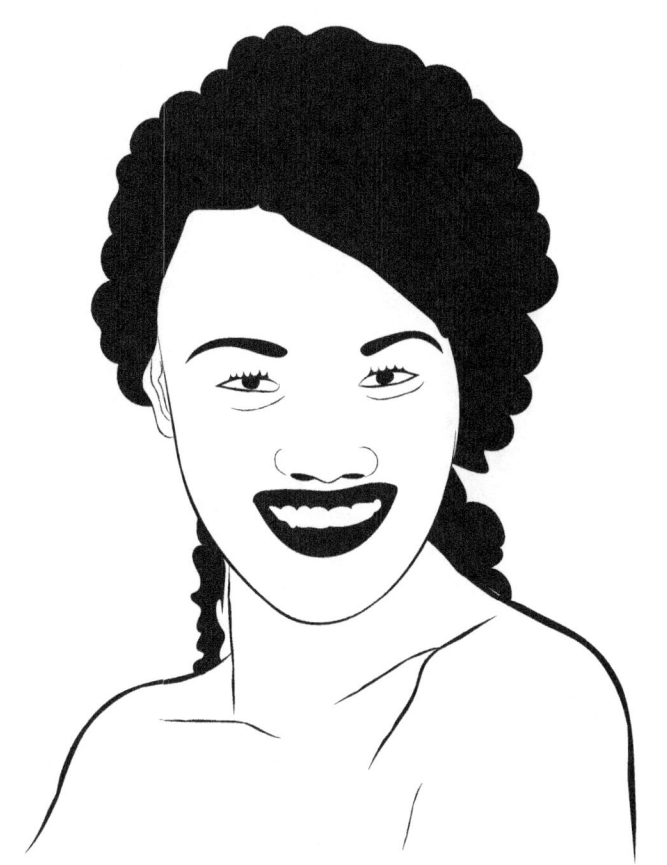

GIRLS MIGHT EXCEL IN SOCIAL AND
EMOTIONAL LEARNING PROGRAMS.

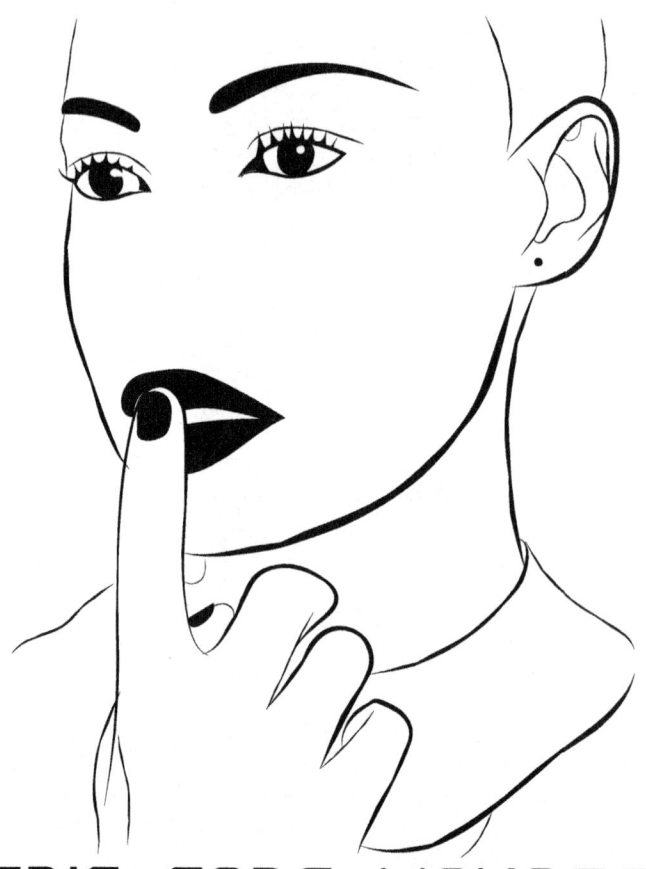

GERIATRIC CARE MANAGEMENT:
WOMEN OFTEN SPECIALIZE IN
CARING FOR ELDERLY INDIVIDUALS.

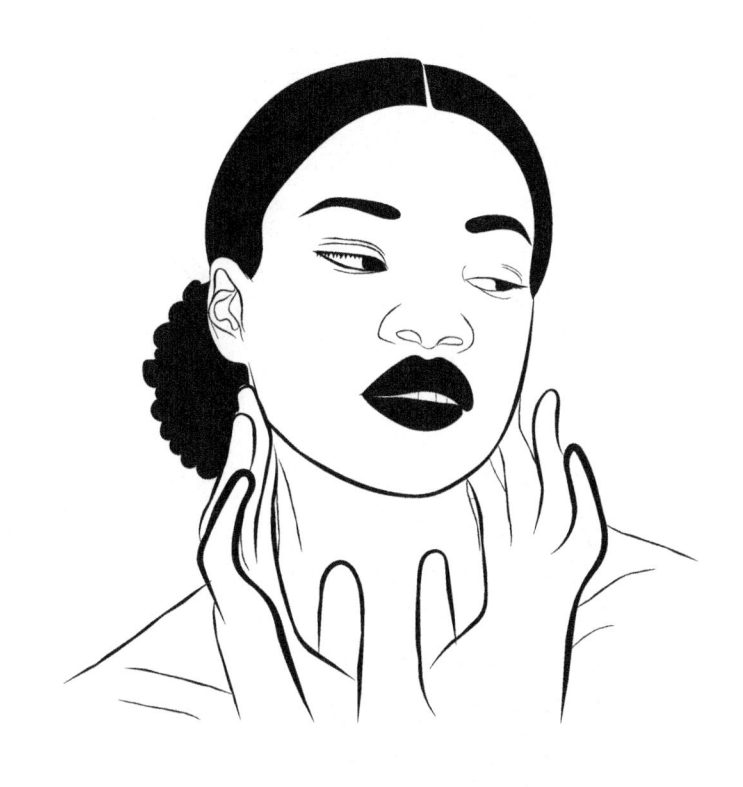

COSMETIC INDUSTRY: WOMEN ARE LEADERS IN THE COSMETICS AND BEAUTY INDUSTRY.

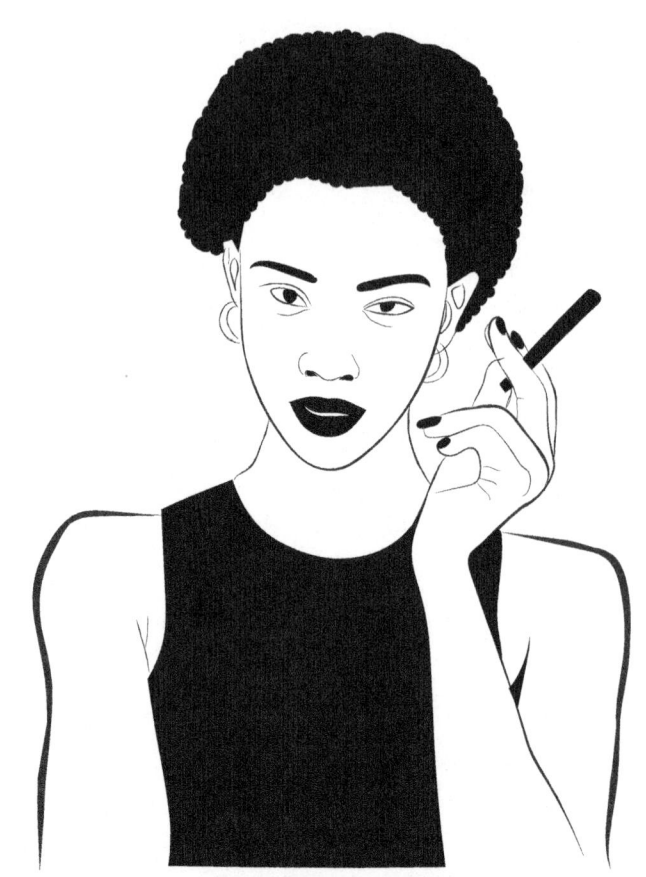

VETERINARY MEDICINE: WOMEN ARE INCREASINGLY PREVALENT IN VETERINARY MEDICINE.

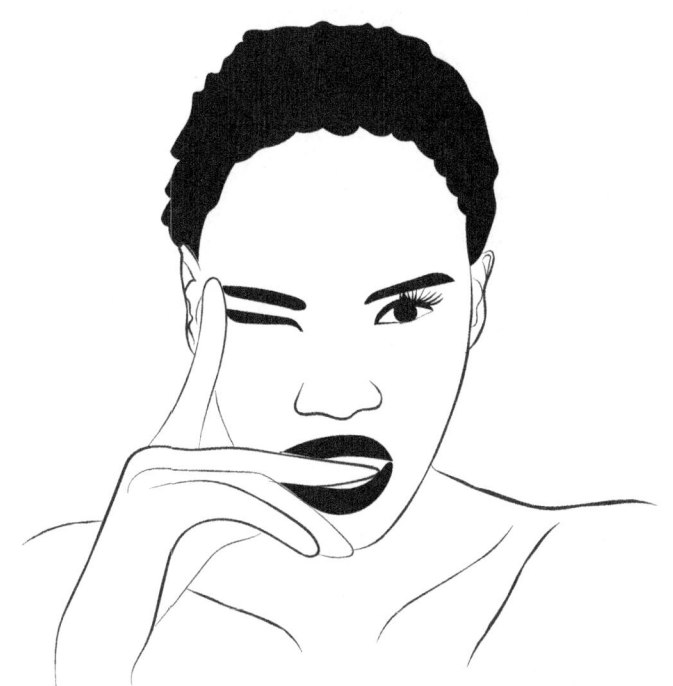

COMMUNITY DEVELOPMENT: WOMEN PLAY VITAL ROLES IN COMMUNITY DEVELOPMENT PROJECTS.

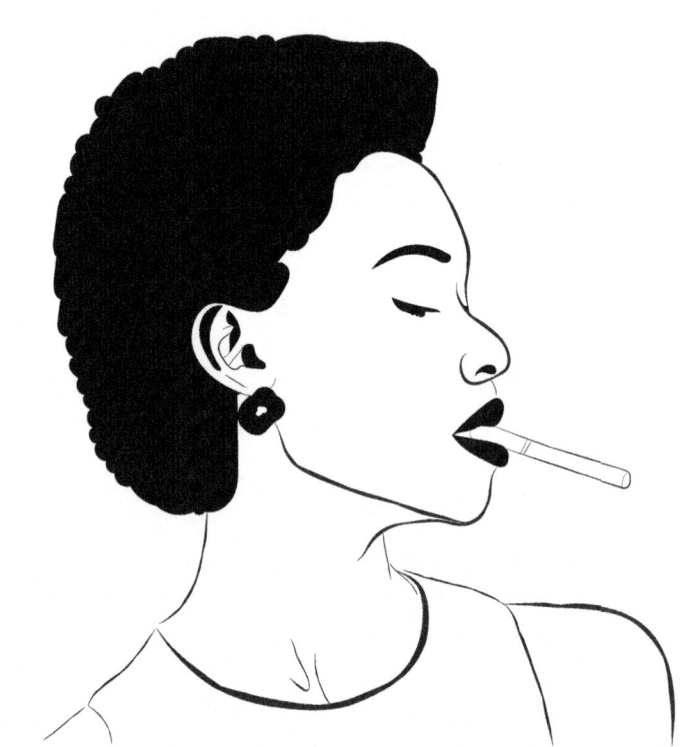

YOGA AND WELLNESS: WOMEN OFTEN LEAD YOGA AND WELLNESS PRACTICES.

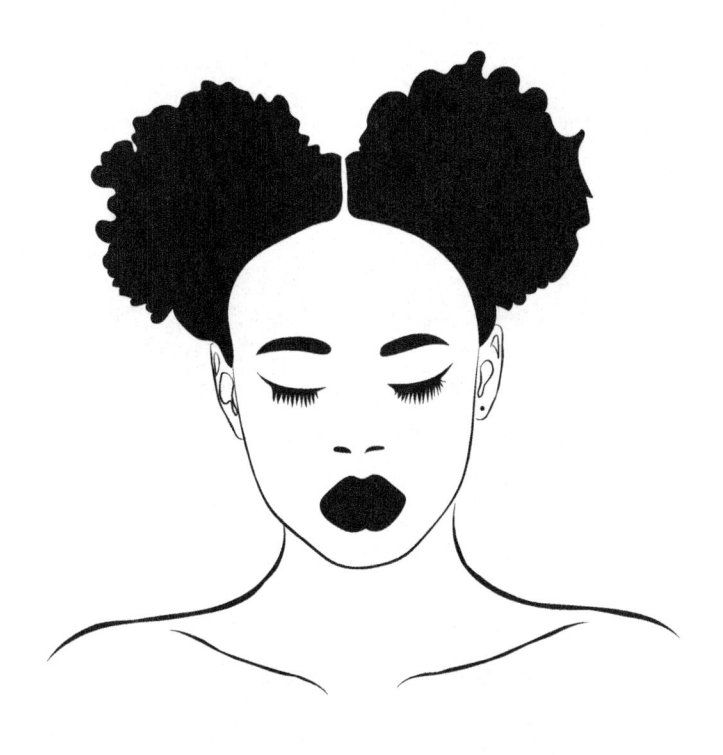

HOSPITALITY AND TOURISM: WOMEN EXCEL IN THE HOSPITALITY INDUSTRY.

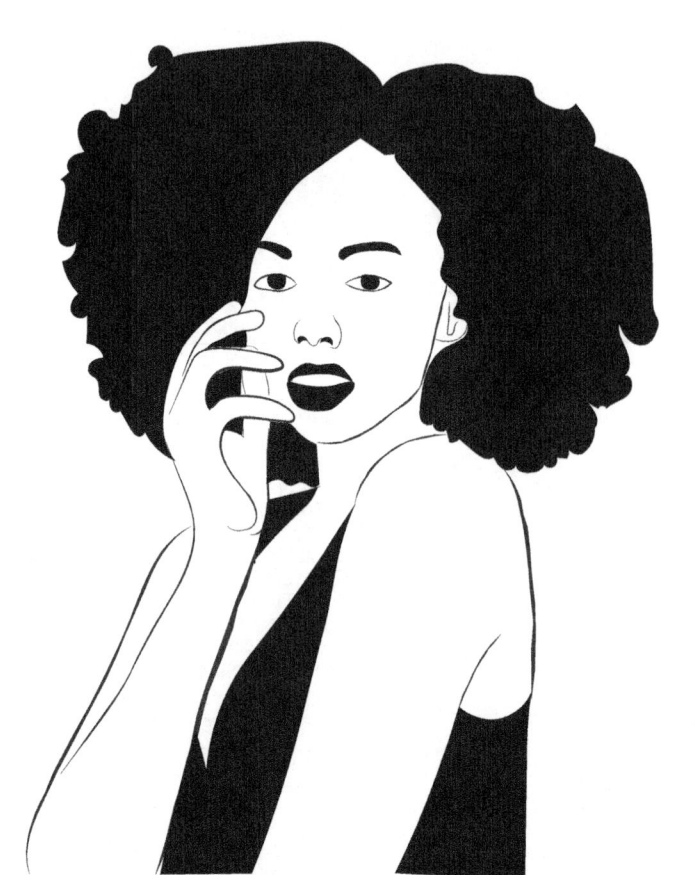

TEXTILE DESIGN: WOMEN OFTEN WORK AS TEXTILE DESIGNERS.

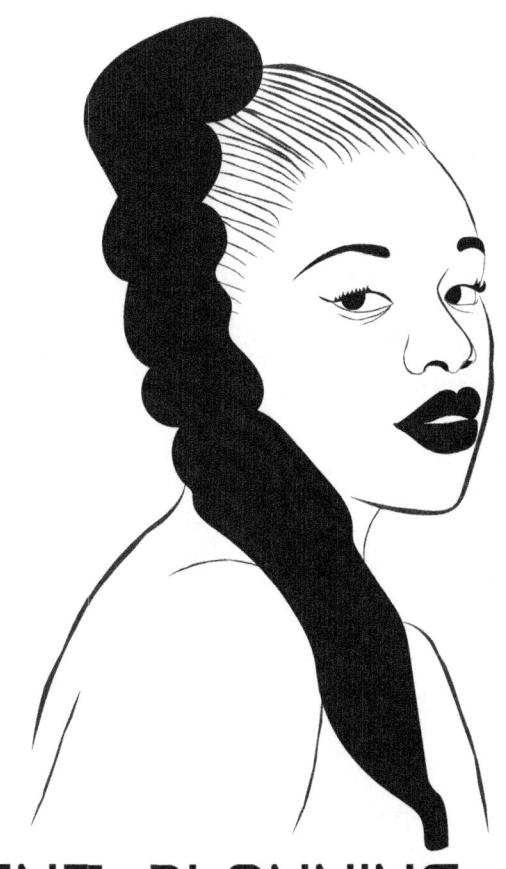

EVENT PLANNING: MANY SUCCESSFUL EVENT PLANNERS ARE WOMEN.

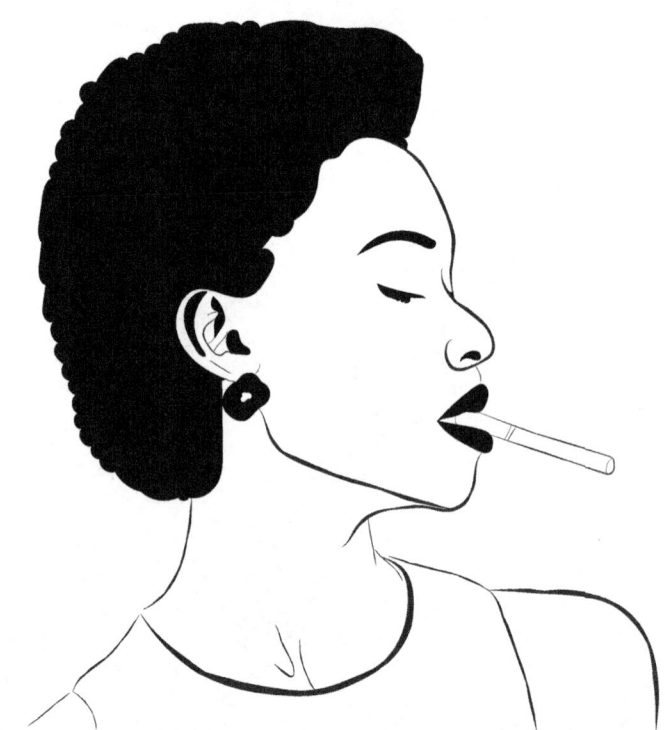

PUBLIC RELATIONS: WOMEN ARE PROMINENT IN PUBLIC RELATIONS ROLES.

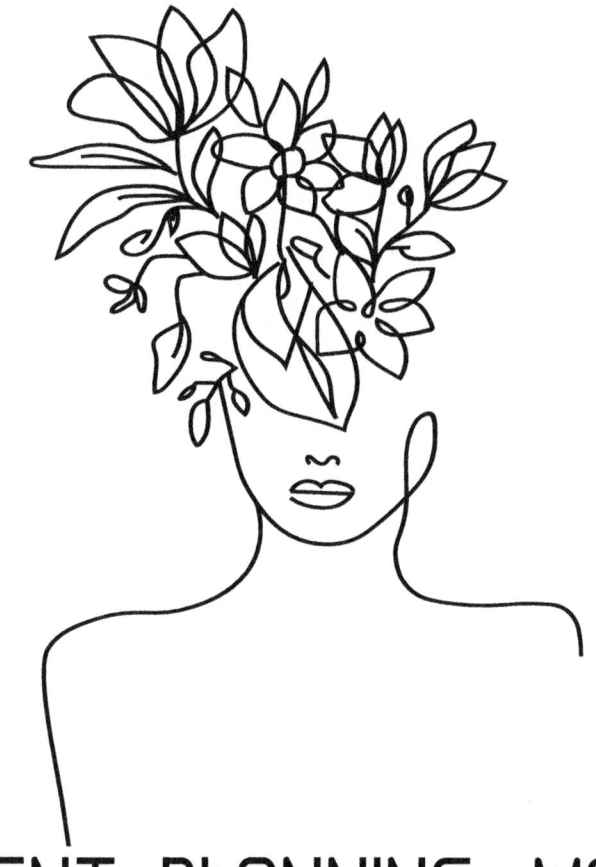

EVENT PLANNING: MANY SUCCESSFUL EVENT PLANNERS ARE WOMEN.

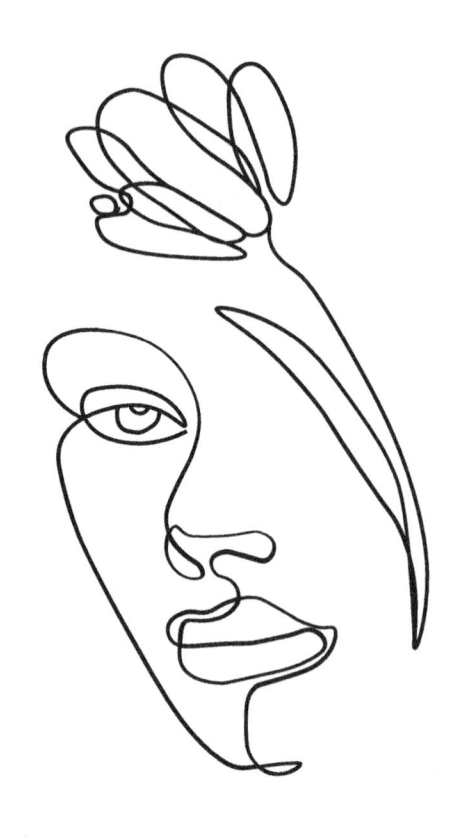

CHILDCARE: WOMEN ARE THE MAJORITY IN CHILDCARE AND EARLY EDUCATION ROLES.

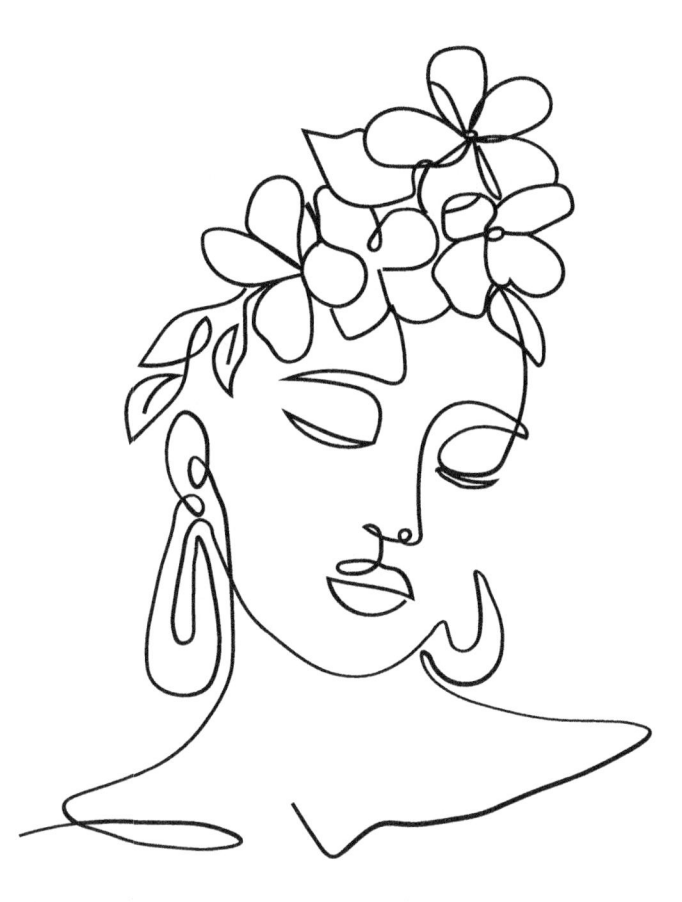

GERONTOLOGY: WOMEN ARE OFTEN AT THE FOREFRONT OF GERONTOLOGY RESEARCH AND CARE.

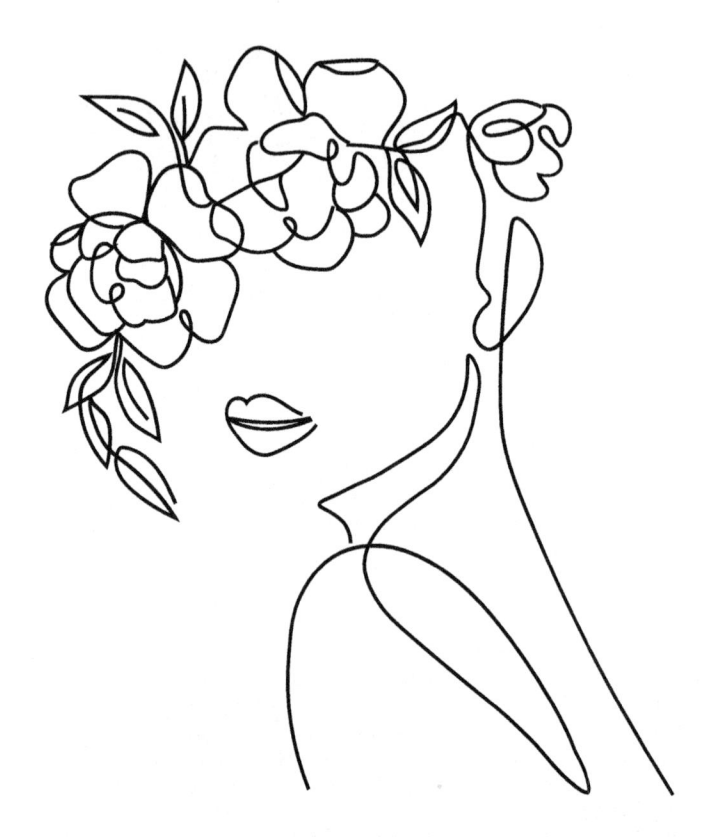

SPEECH-LANGUAGE PATHOLOGY: MANY SPEECH THERAPISTS ARE WOMEN.

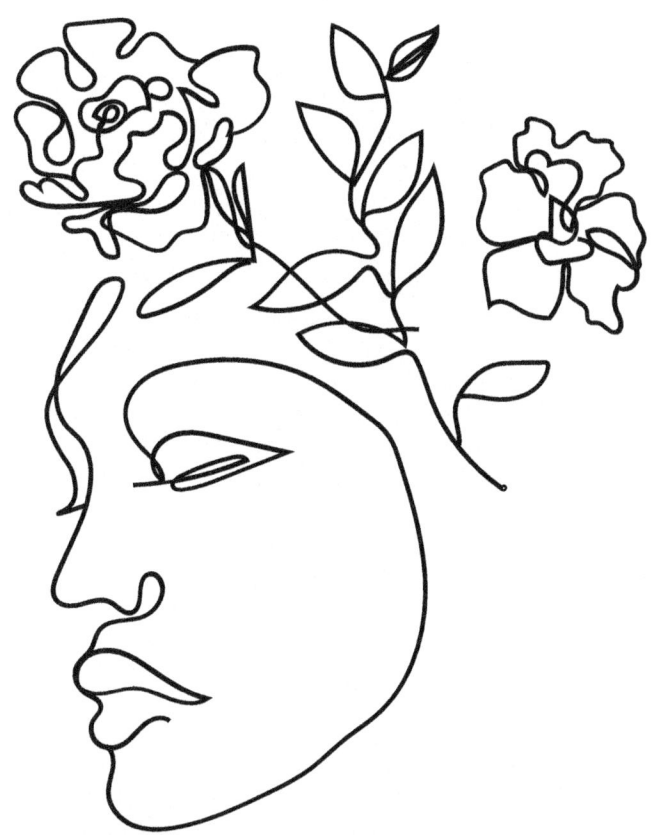

OCCUPATIONAL THERAPY: WOMEN ARE PROMINENT IN THE FIELD OF OCCUPATIONAL THERAPY.

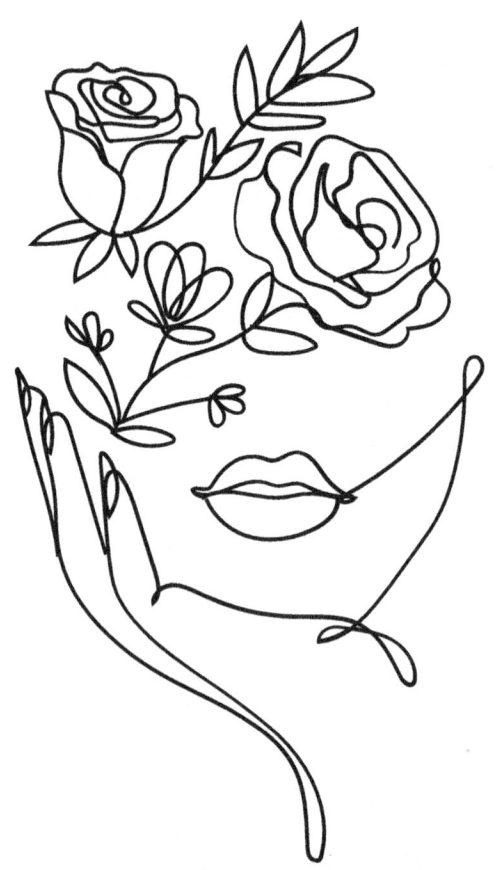

NONPROFIT LEADERSHIP: MANY NONPROFIT ORGANIZATIONS ARE LED BY WOMEN.

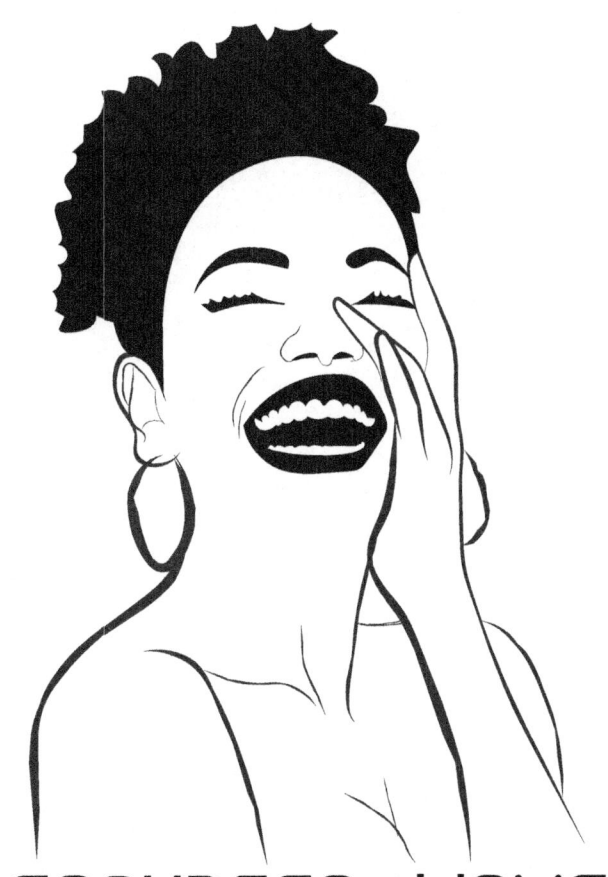

HUMAN RESOURCES: WOMEN OFTEN HOLD KEY ROLES IN HR DEPARTMENTS.

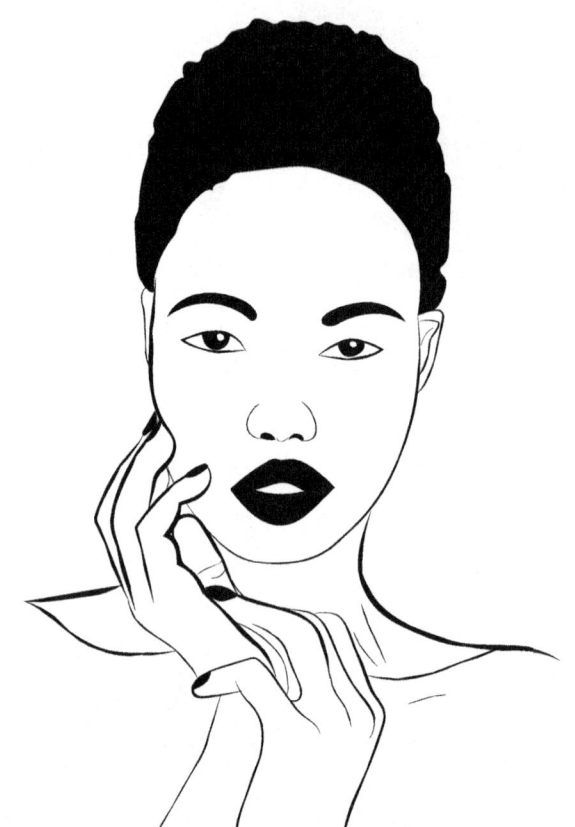

PHILANTHROPY: WOMEN ARE ACTIVELY INVOLVED IN CHARITABLE WORK AND PHILANTHROPY.

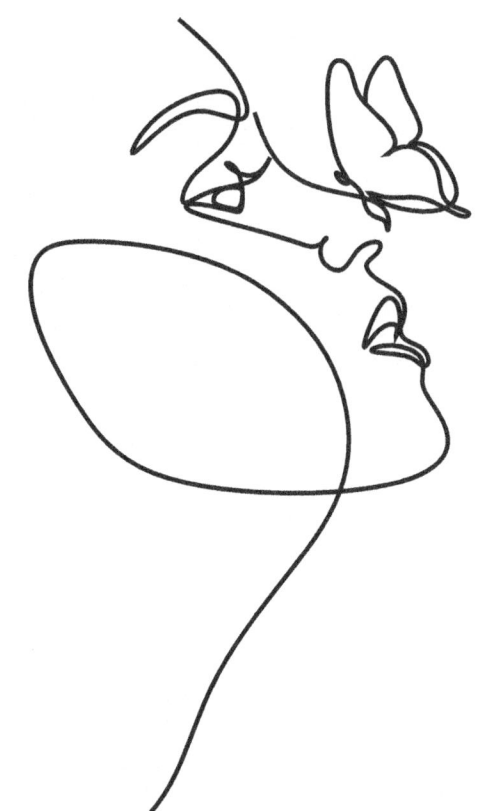

ENVIRONMENTAL CONSERVATION:
MANY WOMEN ARE LEADERS IN
ENVIRONMENTAL ACTIVISM AND
CONSERVATION.

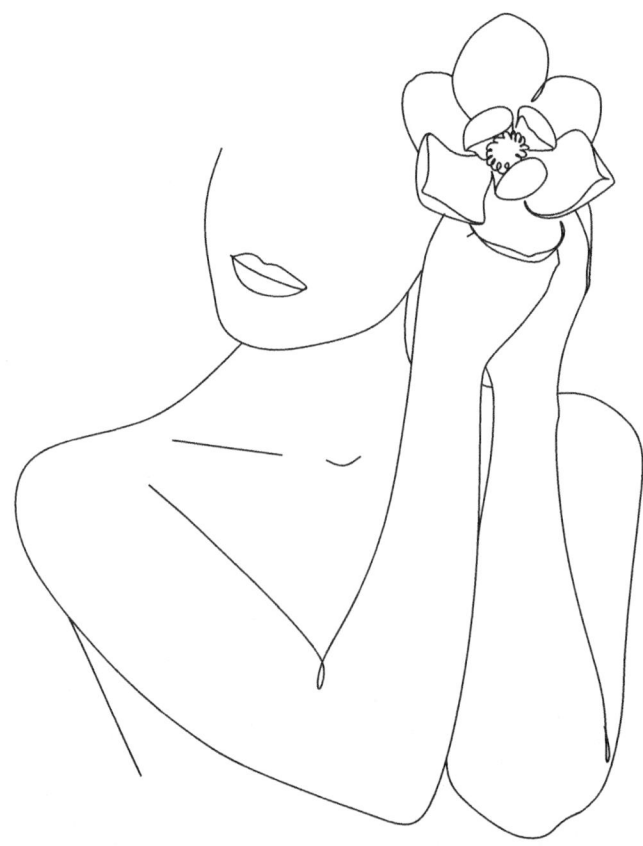

LITERATURE AND WRITING: WOMEN AUTHORS HAVE MADE SUBSTANTIAL CONTRIBUTIONS TO LITERATURE.

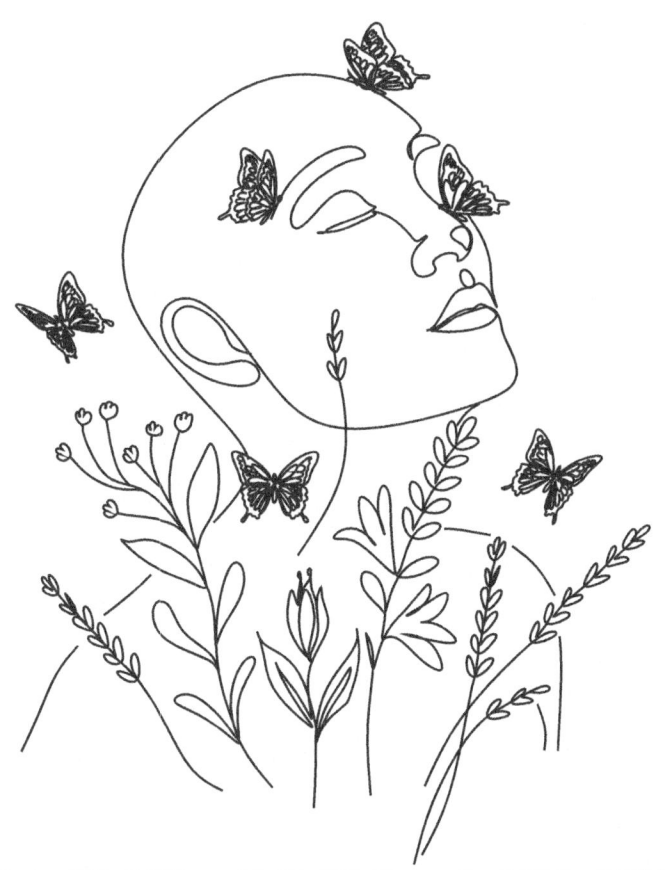

PERFORMING ARTS: WOMEN EXCEL AS ACTORS, DANCERS, AND MUSICIANS.

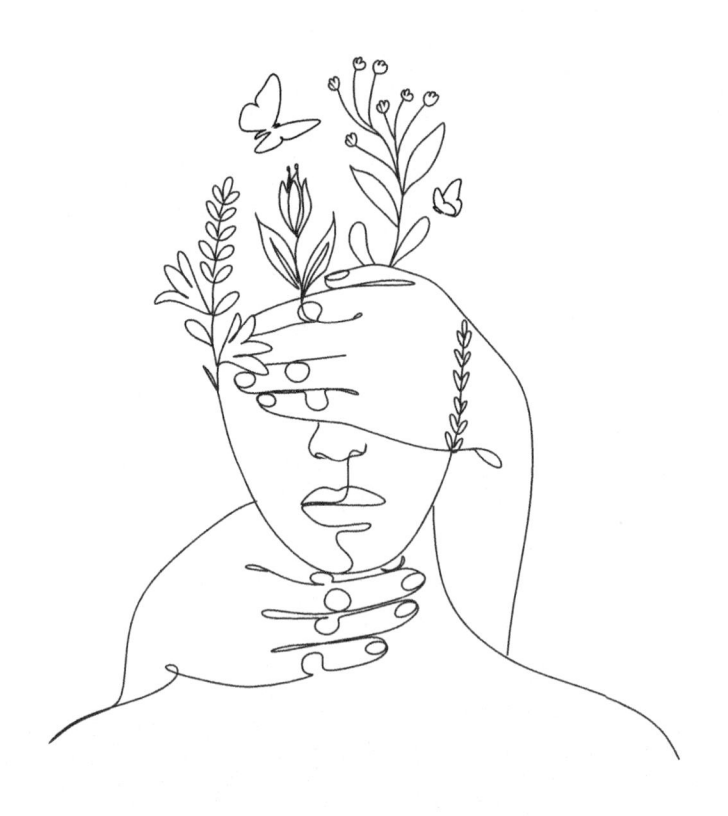

LIBRARY SCIENCE: WOMEN HAVE HISTORICALLY BEEN LIBRARIANS AND ARCHIVISTS.

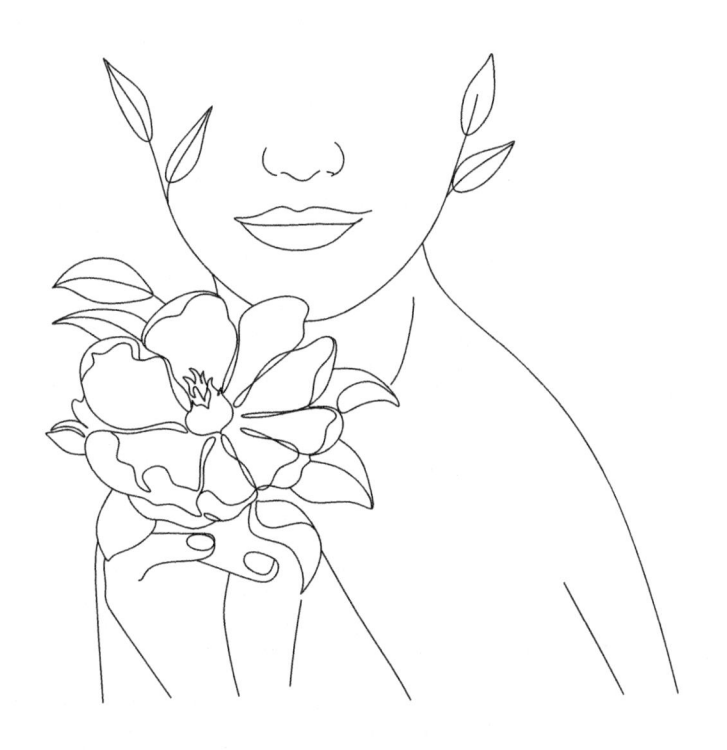

FASHION DESIGN: WOMEN DOMINATE THE FASHION INDUSTRY.

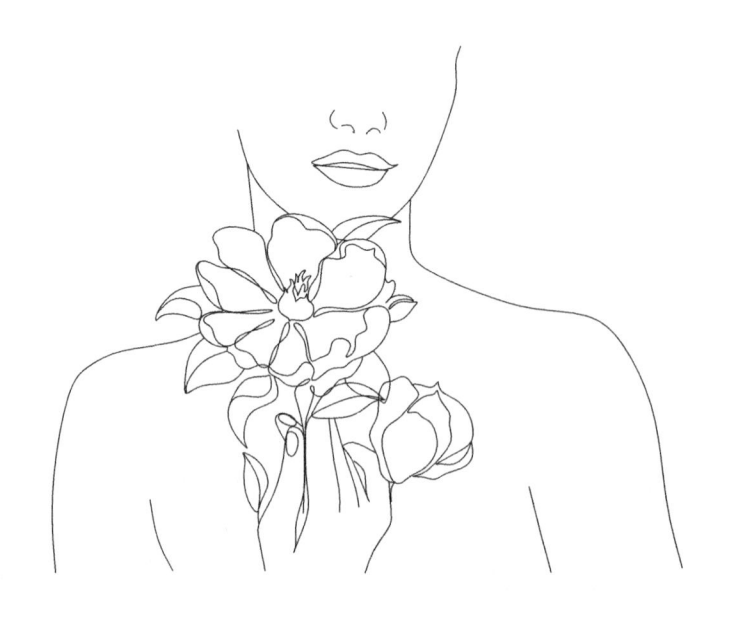

INTERIOR DESIGN: MANY SUCCESSFUL INTERIOR DESIGNERS ARE WOMEN.

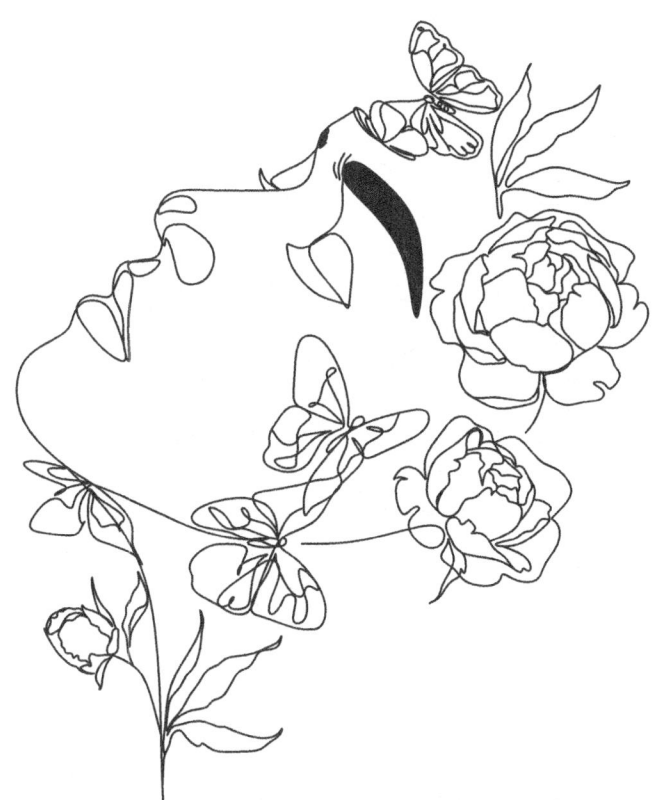

PUBLIC HEALTH: WOMEN HAVE CONTRIBUTED SIGNIFICANTLY TO PUBLIC HEALTH INITIATIVES.

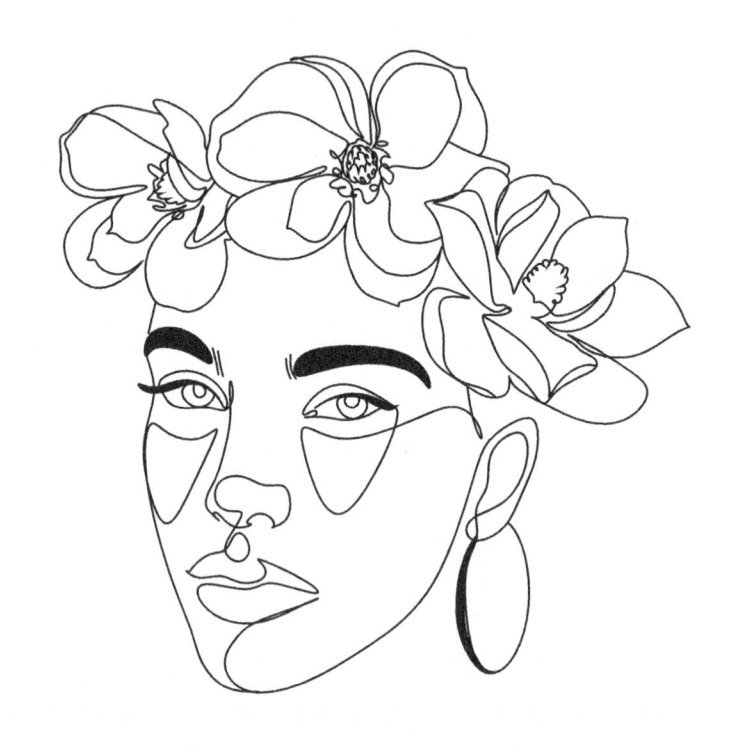

SOCIAL WORK: WOMEN ARE PROMINENT IN SOCIAL WORK AND HUMAN SERVICES.

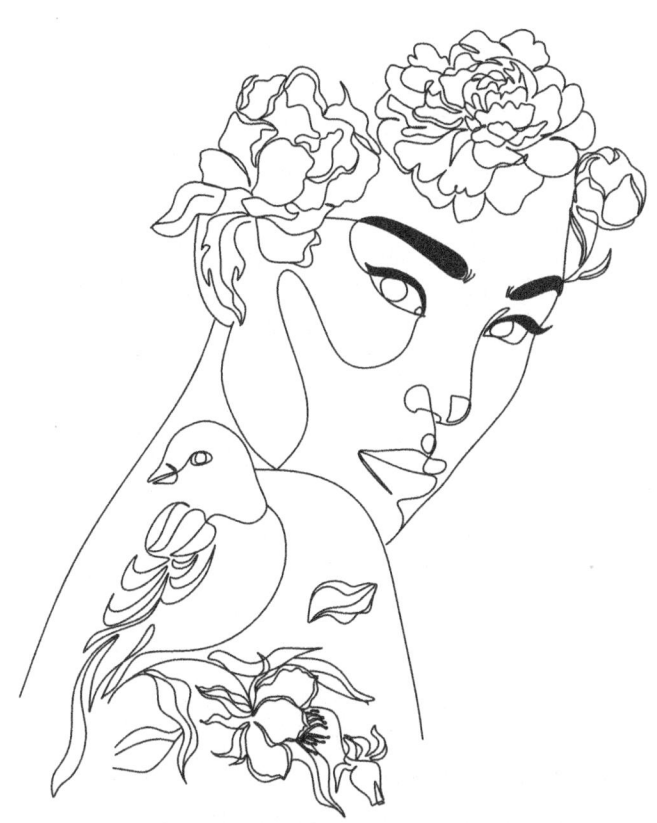

NUTRITION AND DIETETICS: WOMEN OFTEN WORK AS NUTRITIONISTS AND DIETITIANS.

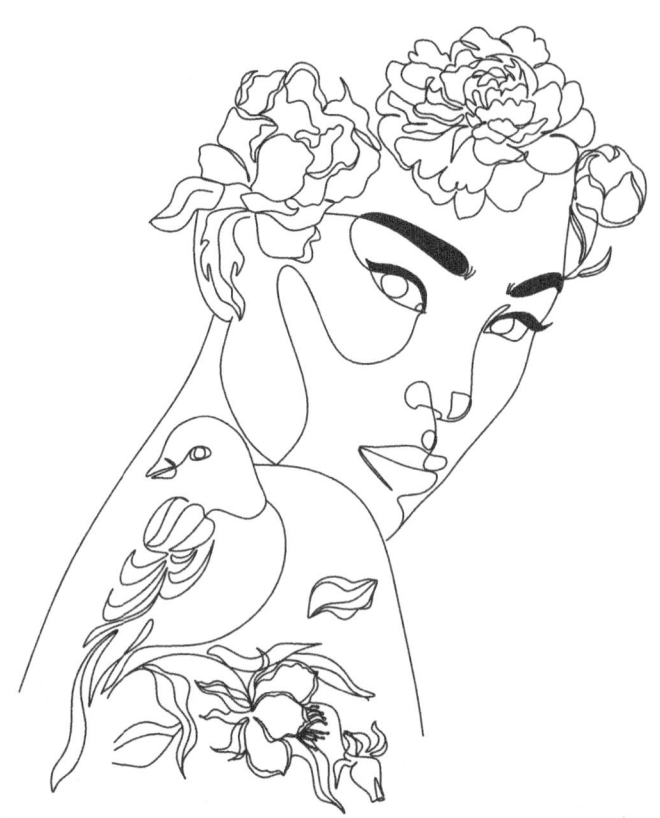

NUTRITION AND DIETETICS: WOMEN OFTEN WORK AS NUTRITIONISTS AND DIETITIANS.

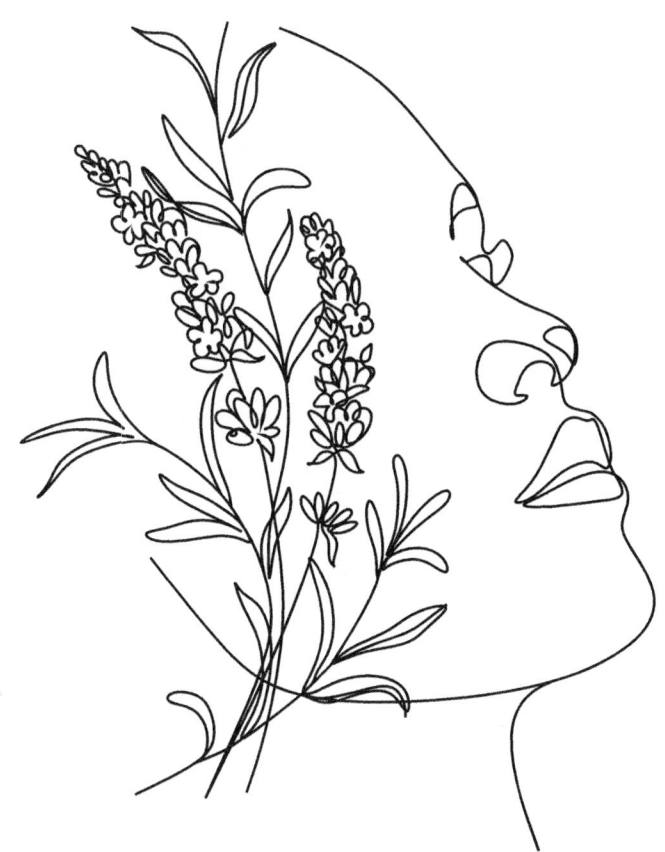

PSYCHOLOGY: MANY PIONEERING PSYCHOLOGISTS HAVE BEEN WOMEN.

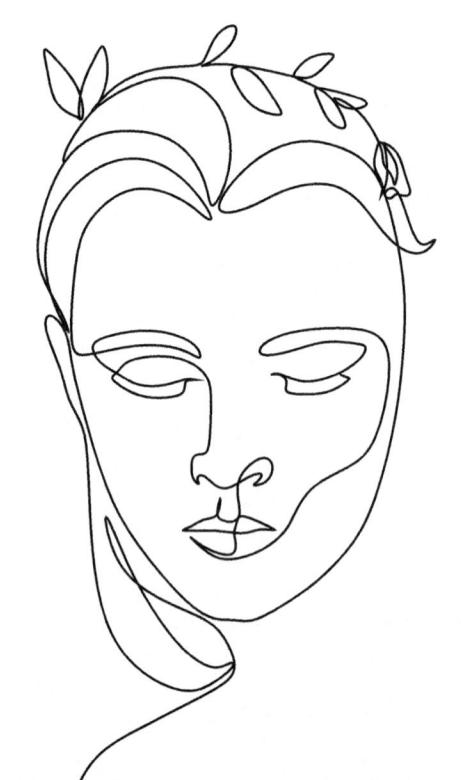

EDUCATION: WOMEN HAVE TRADITIONALLY BEEN LEADERS IN THE FIELD OF EDUCATION.

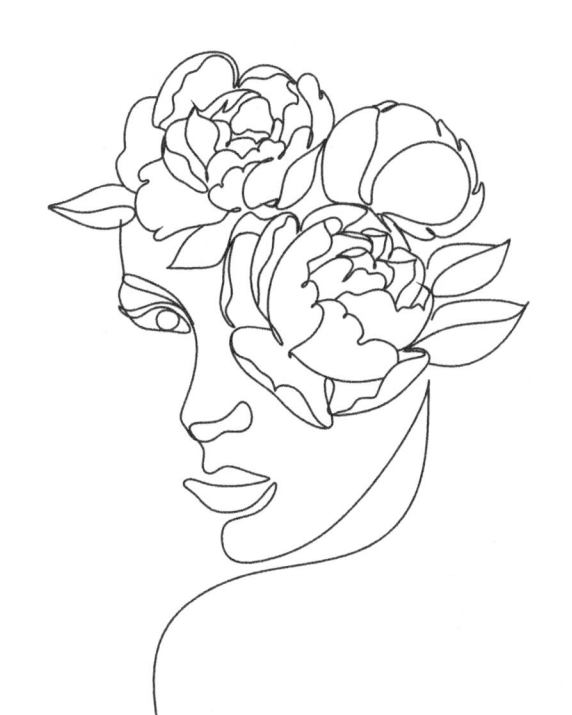

NURSING: NURSING IS A
PREDOMINANTLY FEMALE FIELD,
WITH MANY WOMEN PROVIDING
CRITICAL CARE.

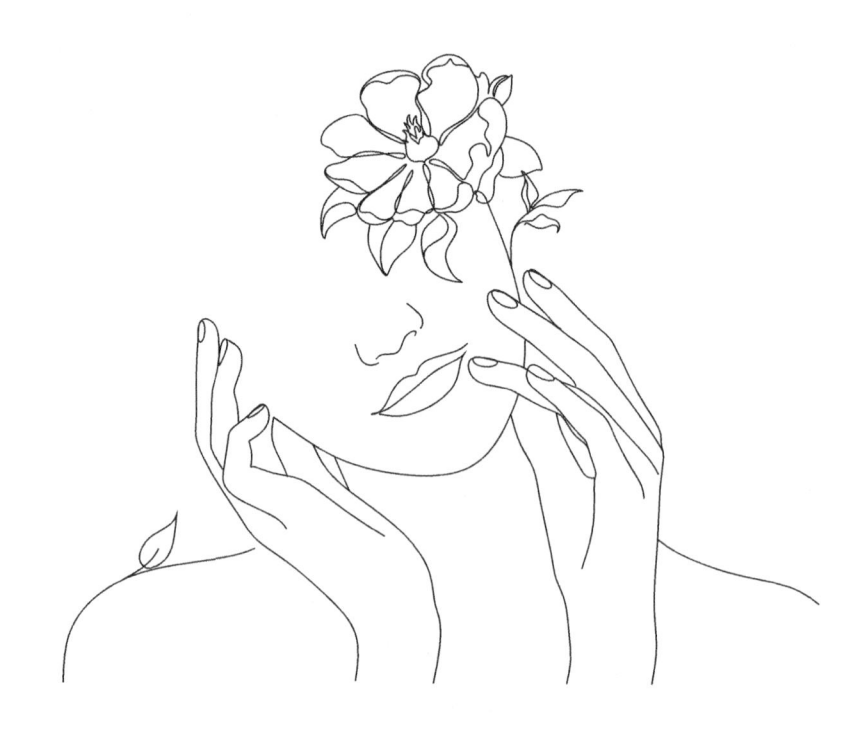

MEDICINE: WOMEN EXCEL IN MEDICAL FIELDS, CONTRIBUTING TO ADVANCEMENTS IN HEALTHCARE AND RESEARCH.

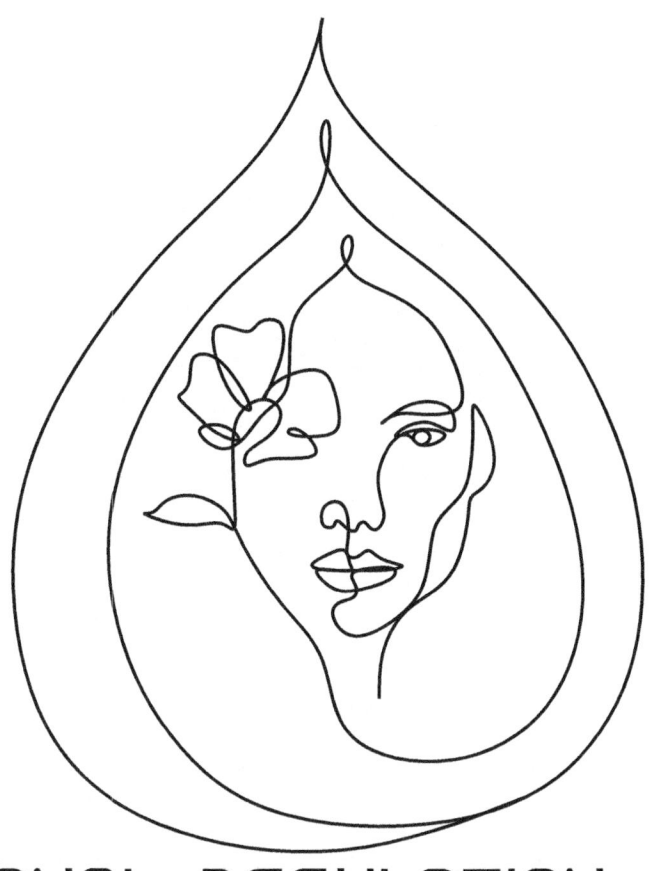

EMOTIONAL REGULATION: GIRLS MAY HAVE BETTER EMOTIONAL REGULATION, LEADING TO ENHANCED FOCUS ON STUDIES.

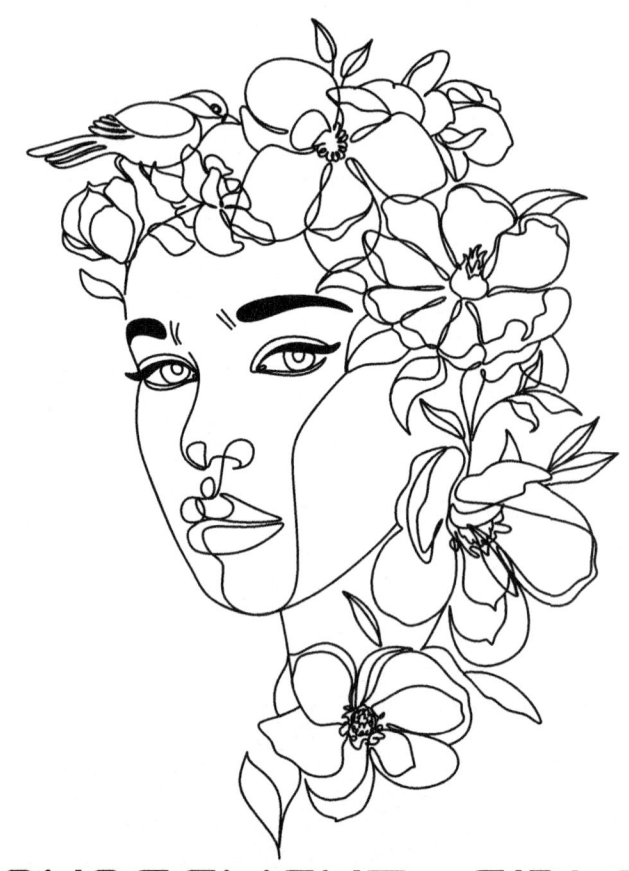

TIME MANAGEMENT: GIRLS HAVE STRONG TIME MANAGEMENT SKILLS FOR BALANCING STUDIES AND OTHER ACTIVITIES.

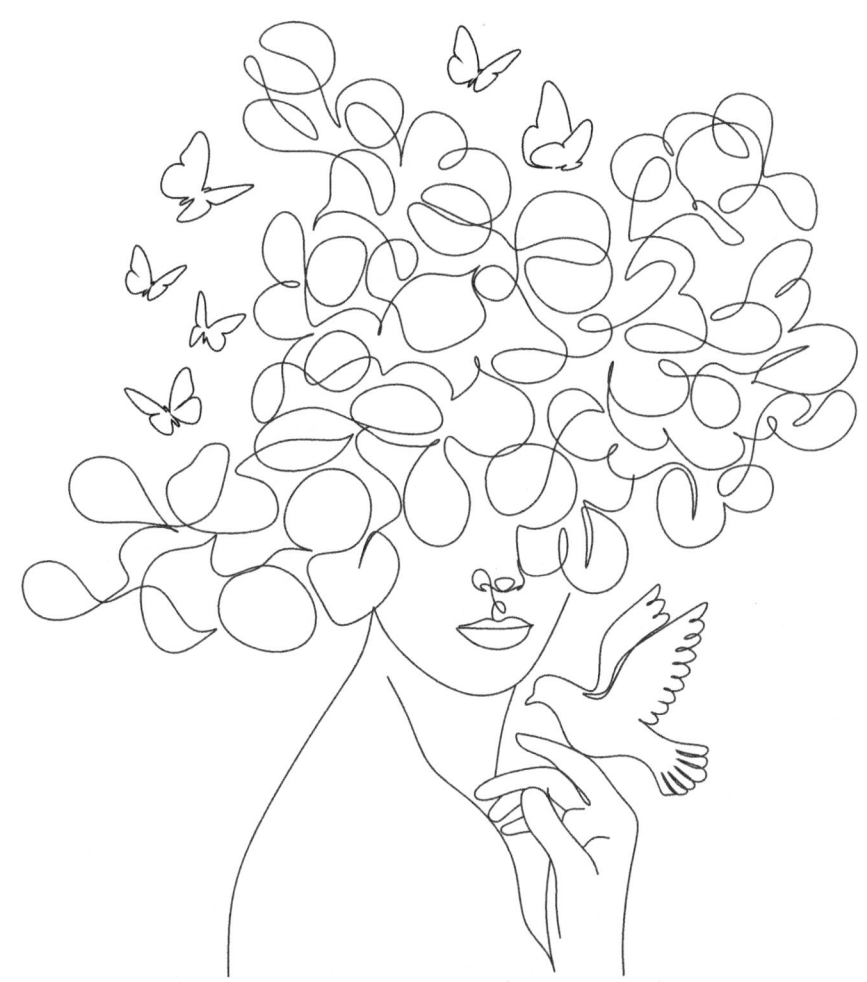

STRESS MANAGEMENT: GIRLS OFTEN MANAGE ACADEMIC STRESS EFFECTIVELY.

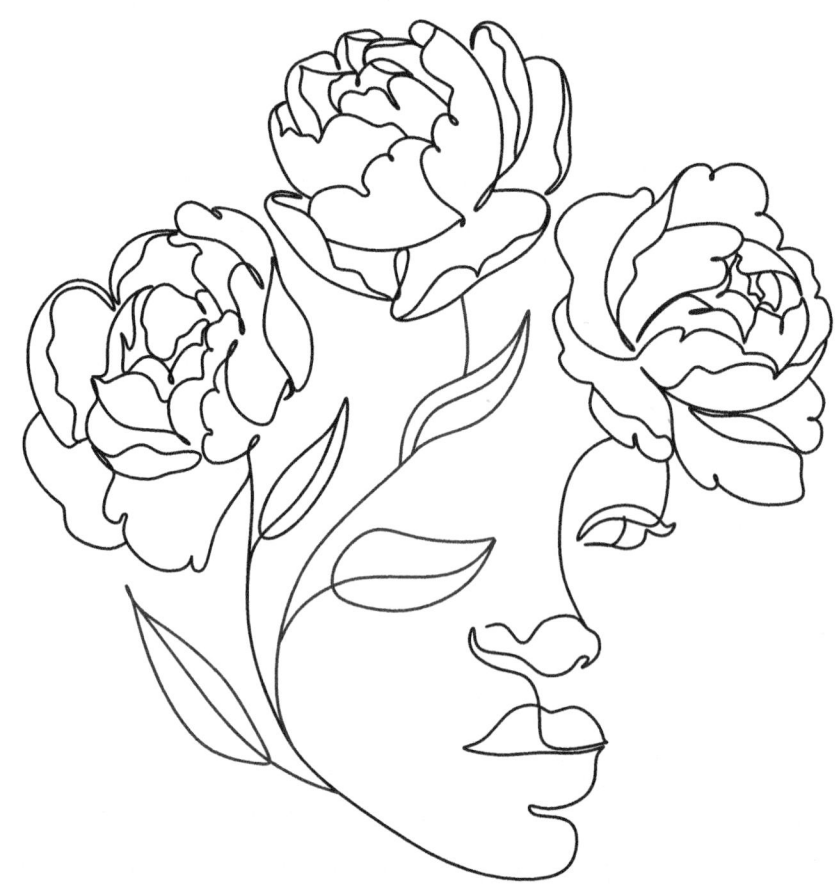

EFFECTIVE NOTE-TAKING: GIRLS EMPLOY EFFECTIVE NOTE-TAKING STRATEGIES.

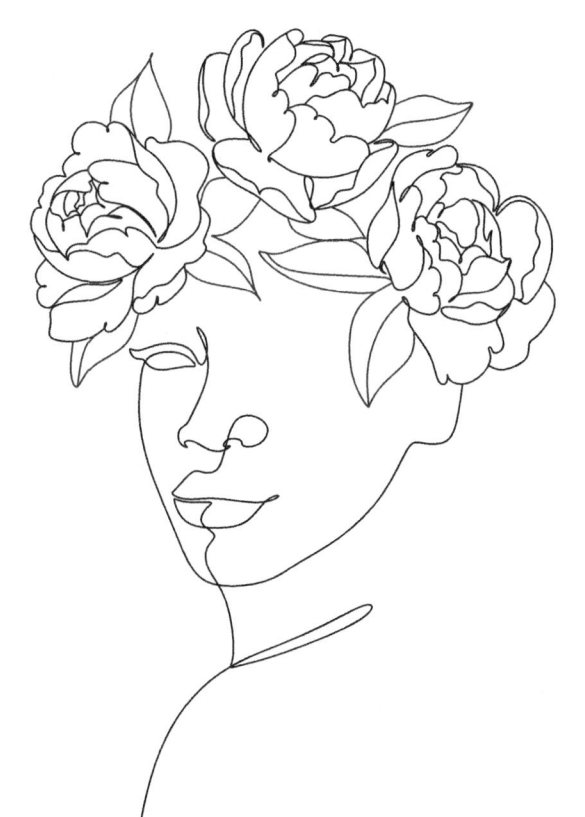

ORGANIZATION OF STUDY MATERIAL: GIRLS TEND TO KEEP THEIR STUDY MATERIALS WELL-ORGANIZED.

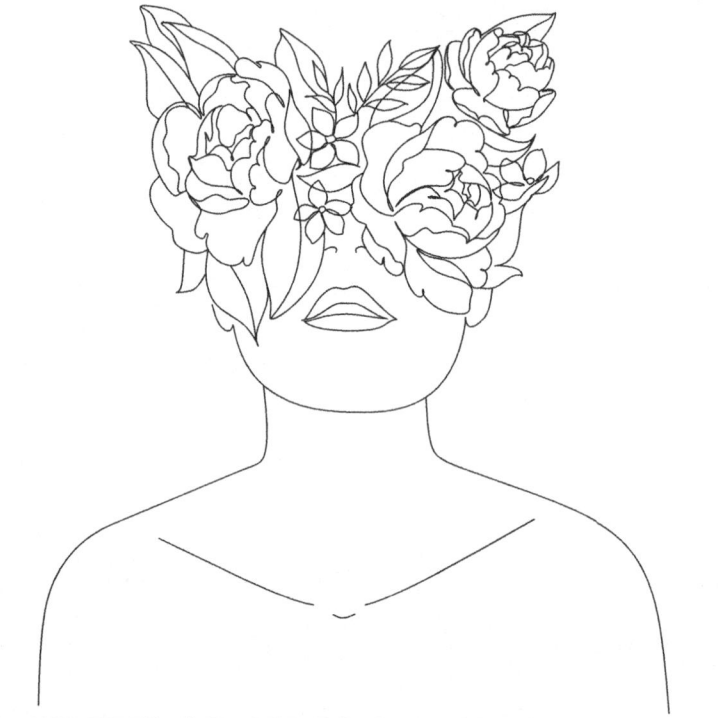

SELF-MOTIVATION: GIRLS MAY BE MORE SELF-MOTIVATED TO ACHIEVE ACADEMIC GOALS.

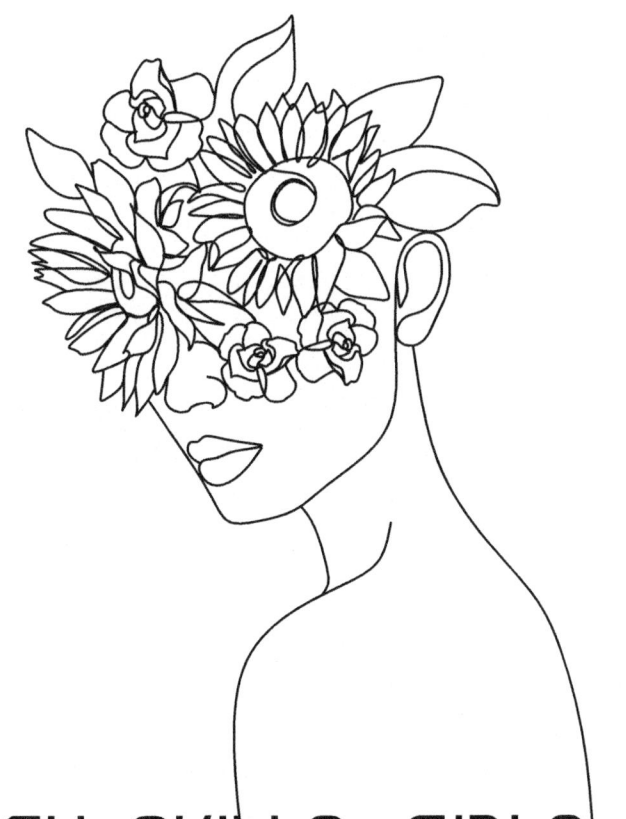

RESEARCH SKILLS: GIRLS OFTEN EXCEL IN RESEARCH AND INFORMATION GATHERING.

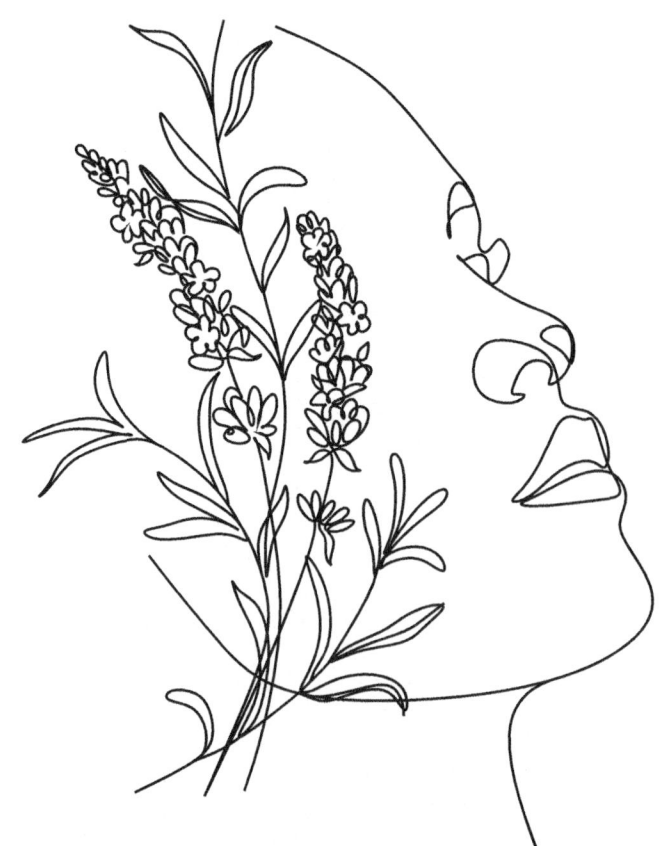

MATHEMATICS: GIRLS CAN PERFORM EQUALLY WELL OR BETTER IN MATHEMATICS, DEPENDING ON THE CONTEXT.

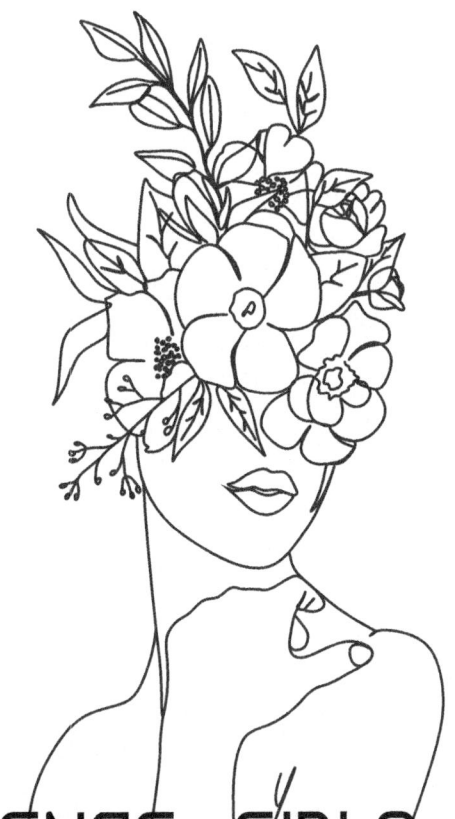

DILIGENCE: GIRLS EXHIBIT
DILIGENCE IN COMPLETING
ASSIGNMENTS AND PROJECTS.

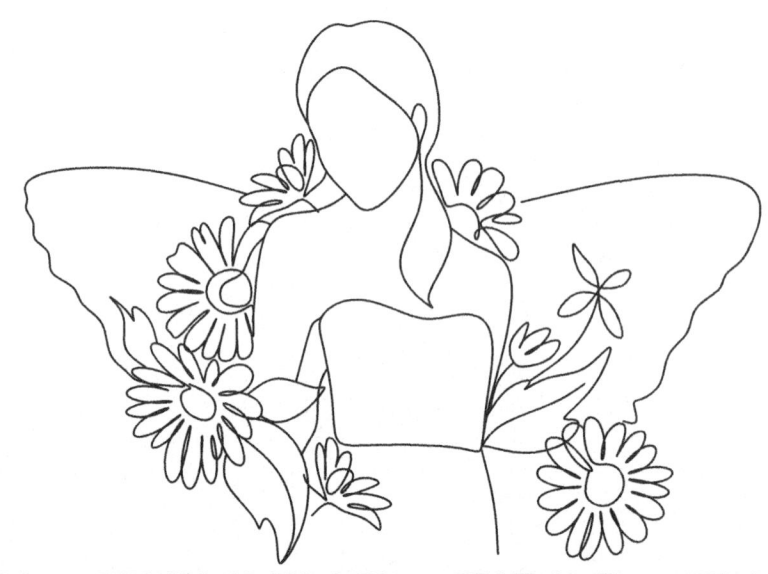

CRITICAL THINKING: GIRLS EXCEL IN CRITICAL THINKING AND PROBLEM-SOLVING SKILLS.

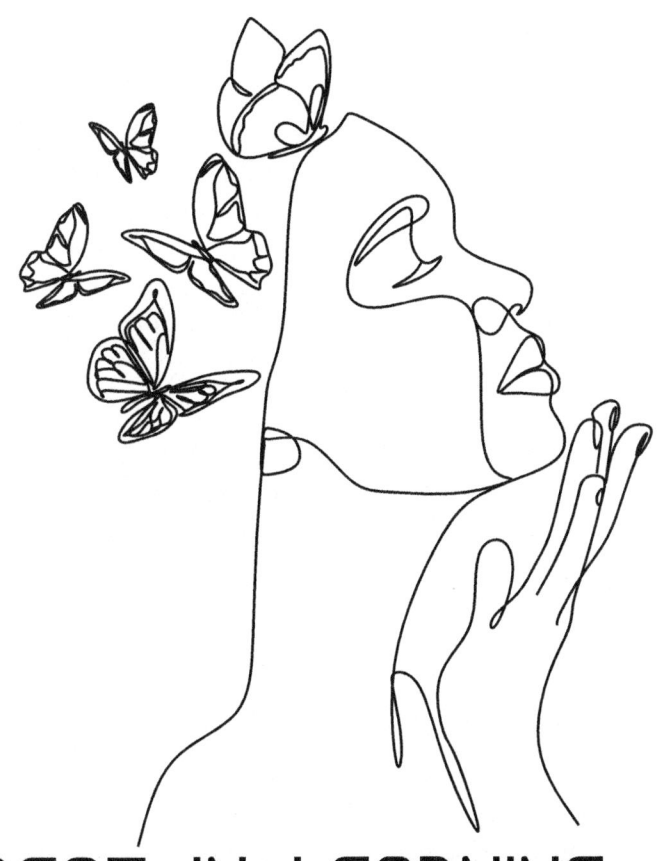

INTEREST IN LEARNING: GIRLS OFTEN EXPRESS A STRONG INTEREST IN LEARNING NEW SUBJECTS.

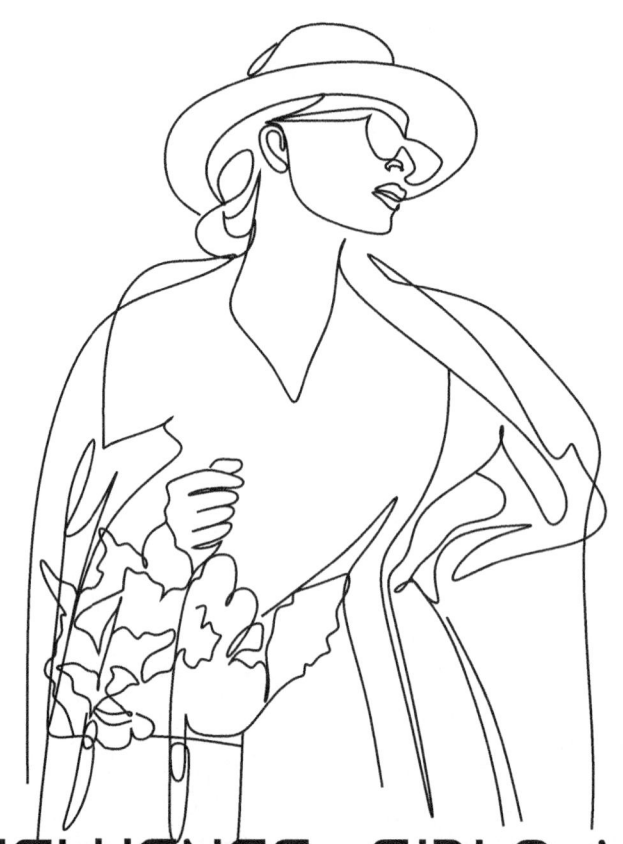

PEER INFLUENCE: GIRLS MAY BE LESS INFLUENCED BY PEER PRESSURE TO UNDERPERFORM ACADEMICALLY.

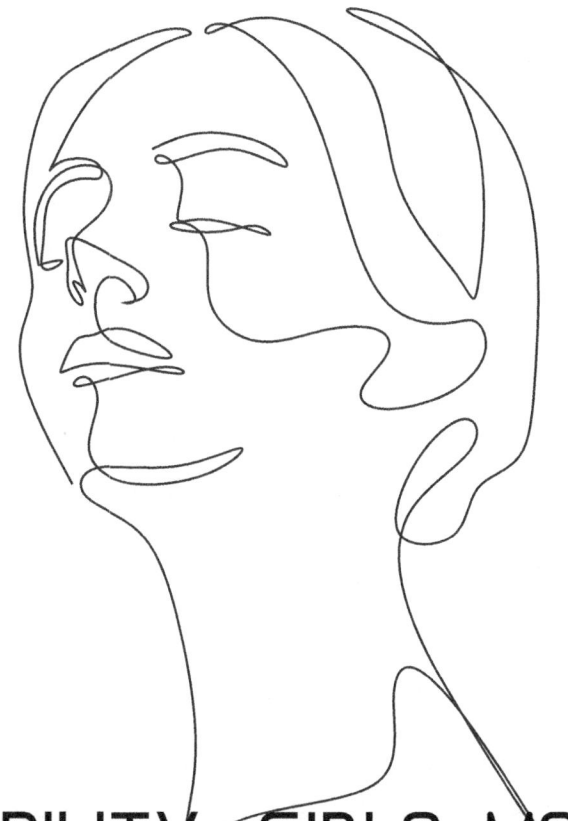

ADAPTABILITY: GIRLS MAY ADAPT MORE EASILY TO CHANGING CLASSROOM ENVIRONMENTS.

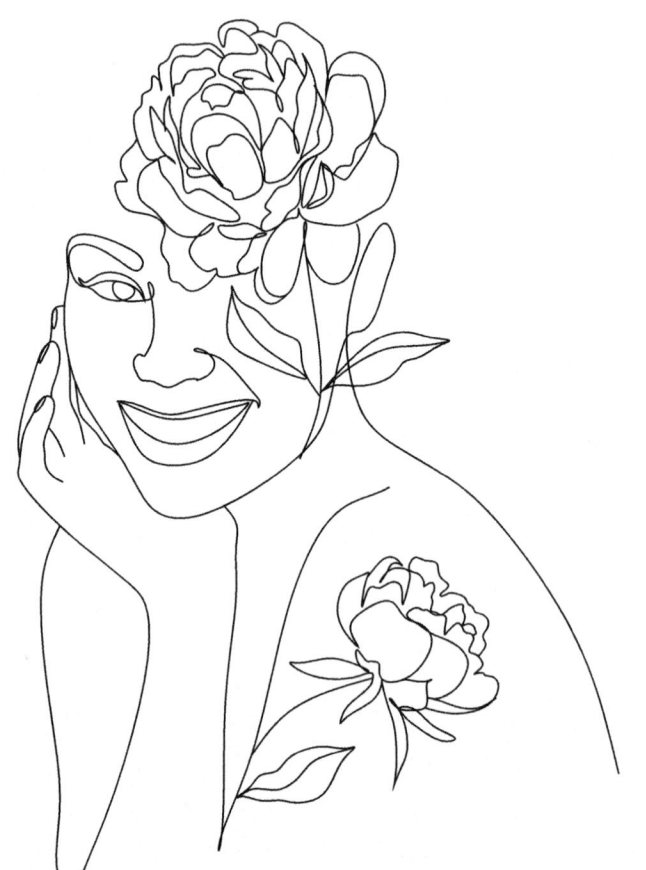

ATTENTION SPAN: GIRLS MAY HAVE LONGER ATTENTION SPANS IN THE CLASSROOM.

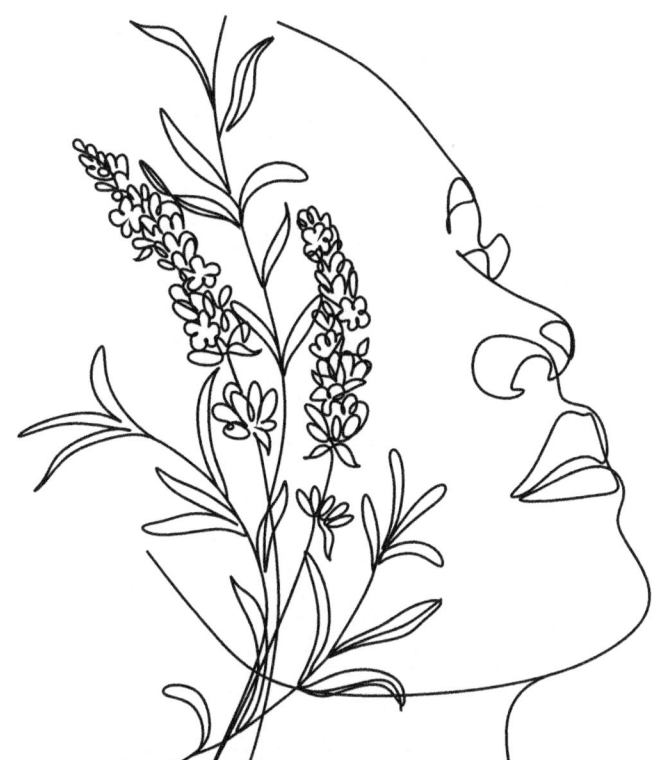

LANGUAGE PROFICIENCY: GIRLS MAY DEMONSTRATE GREATER PROFICIENCY IN LANGUAGES.

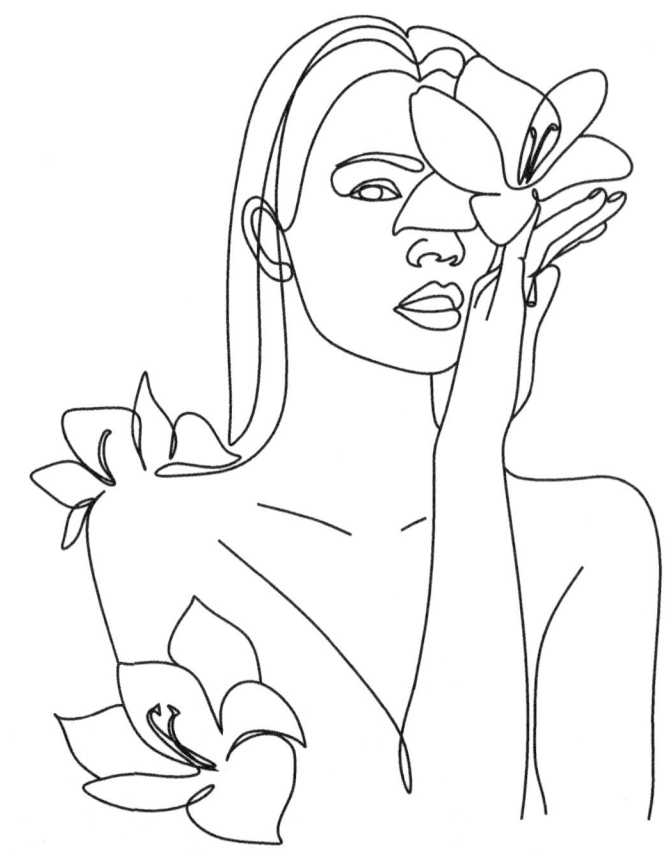

MOTIVATION FOR HIGHER EDUCATION: GIRLS ARE OFTEN MOTIVATED TO PURSUE HIGHER EDUCATION, LEADING TO ACADEMIC SUCCESS.

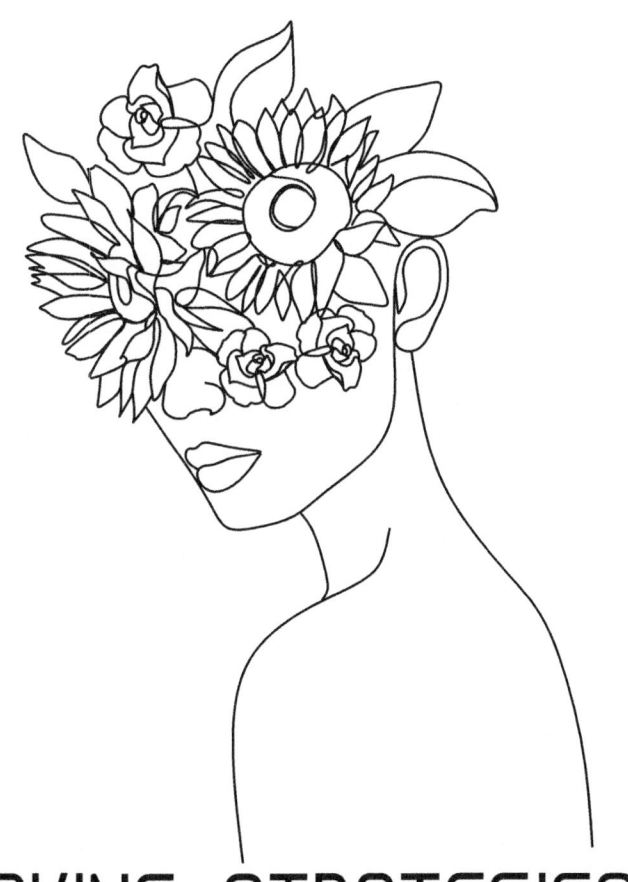

TEST-TAKING STRATEGIES: GIRLS OFTEN EMPLOY EFFECTIVE TEST-TAKING STRATEGIES.

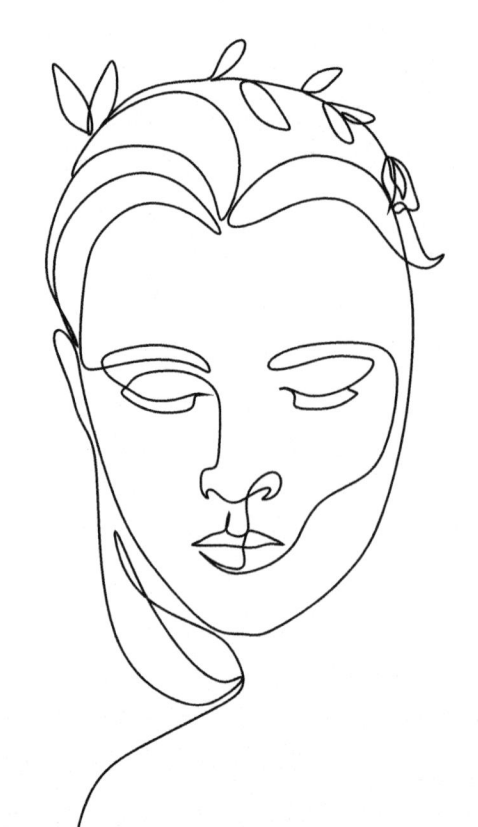

HOMEWORK COMPLETION: GIRLS TEND TO COMPLETE THEIR HOMEWORK ASSIGNMENTS REGULARLY.

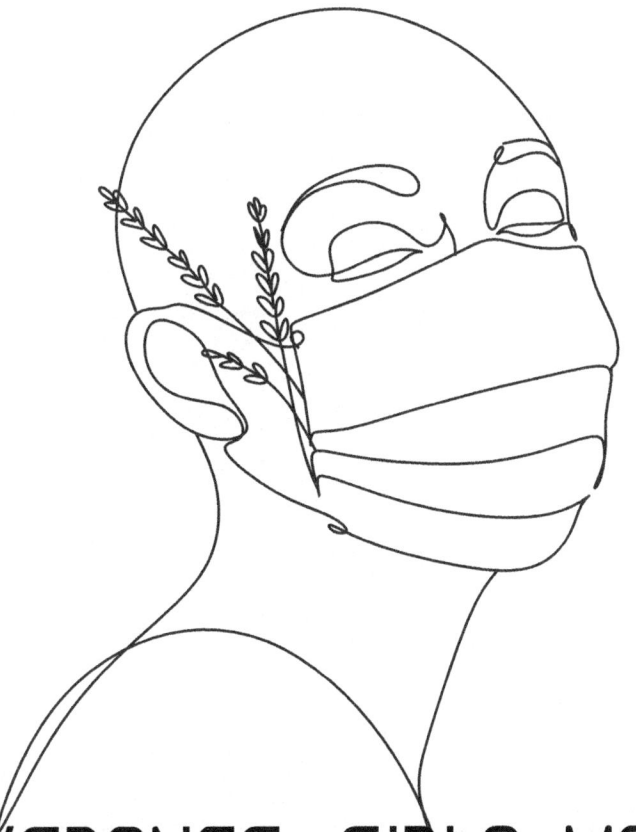

PERSEVERANCE: GIRLS MAY BE MORE PERSISTENT IN TACKLING CHALLENGING SUBJECTS OR ASSIGNMENTS.

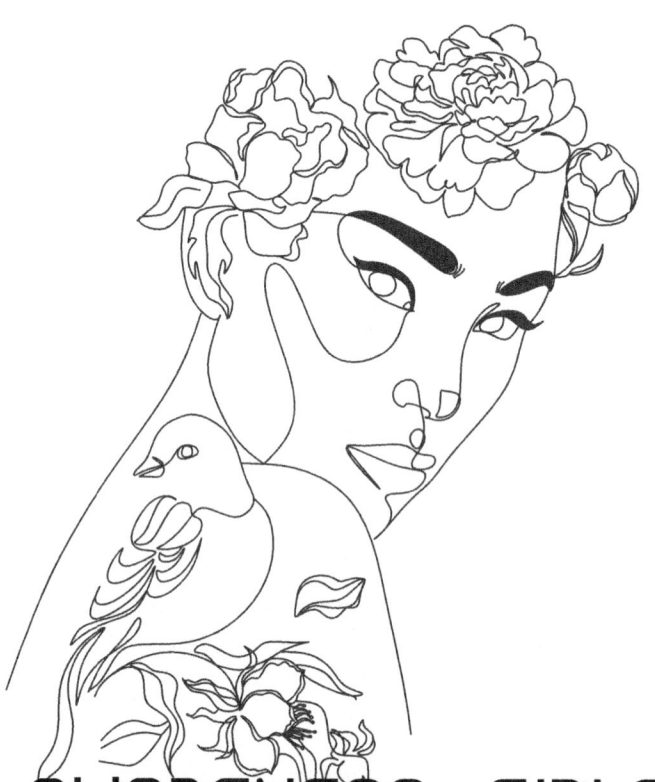

SOCIAL AWARENESS: GIRLS MAY EXCEL IN SUBJECTS THAT REQUIRE AN UNDERSTANDING OF SOCIAL DYNAMICS AND HUMAN BEHAVIOR.

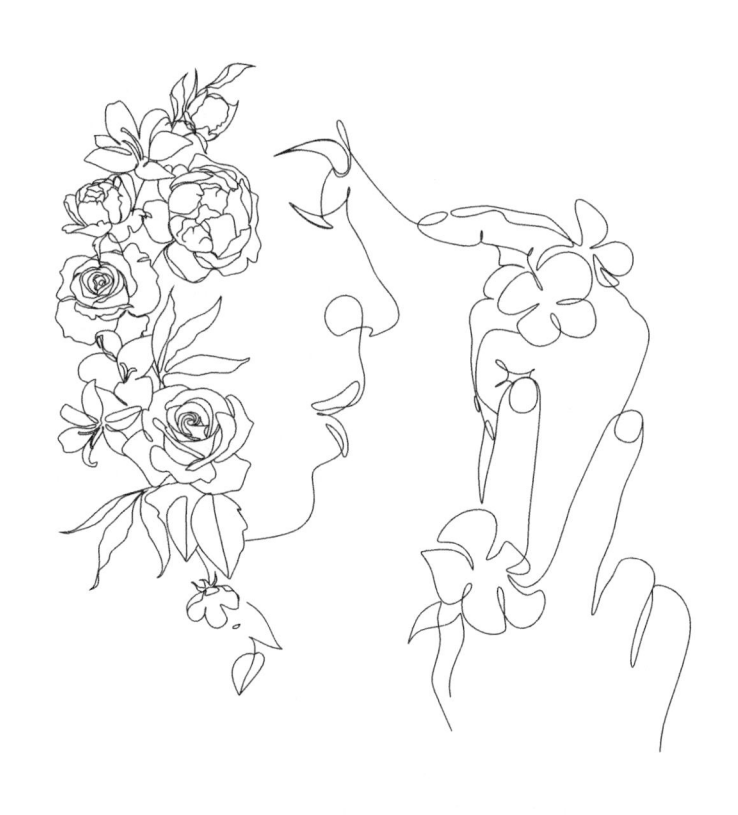

WRITTEN COMMUNICATION: GIRLS OFTEN EXCEL IN WRITTEN COMMUNICATION AND ESSAY WRITING.

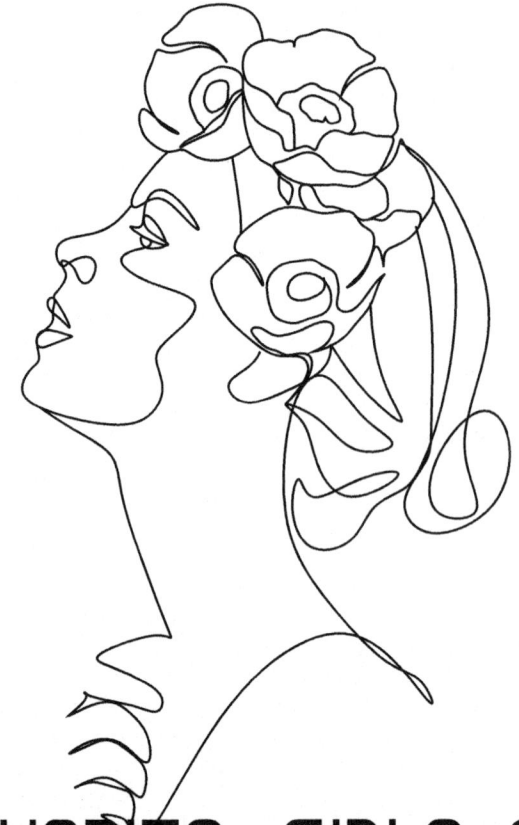

READING HABITS: GIRLS ARE MORE LIKELY TO ENGAGE IN REGULAR READING, WHICH CAN ENHANCE LANGUAGE AND LITERACY SKILLS.

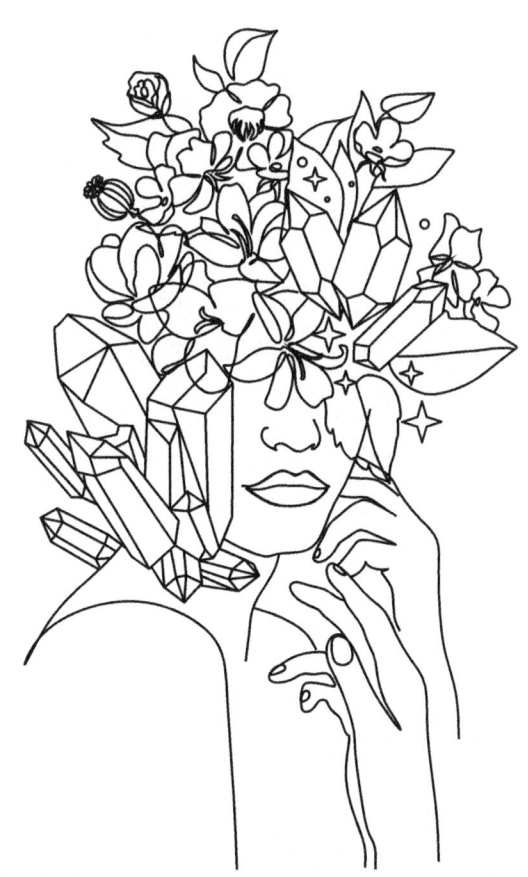

ORGANIZATION: GIRLS ARE OFTEN MORE ORGANIZED, WHICH CAN LEAD TO BETTER STUDY ROUTINES.

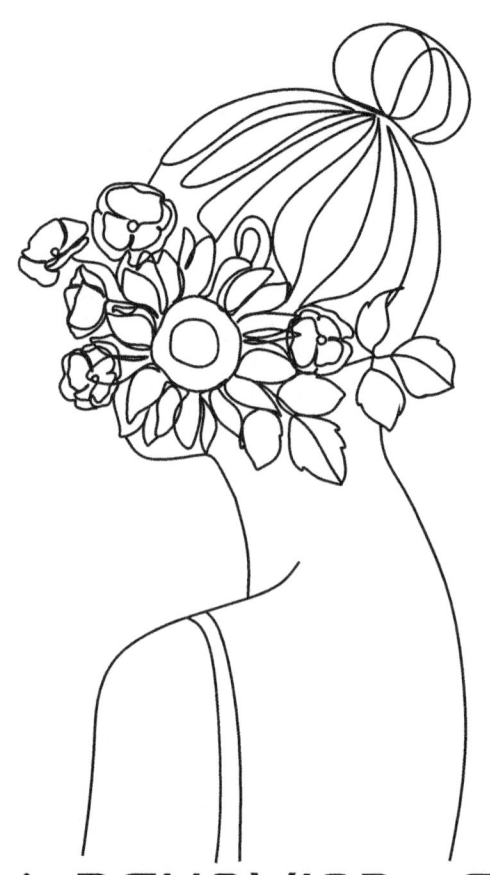

CLASSROOM BEHAVIOR: GIRLS MAY EXHIBIT MORE FAVORABLE CLASSROOM BEHAVIOR, SUCH AS ATTENTIVENESS AND PARTICIPATION.

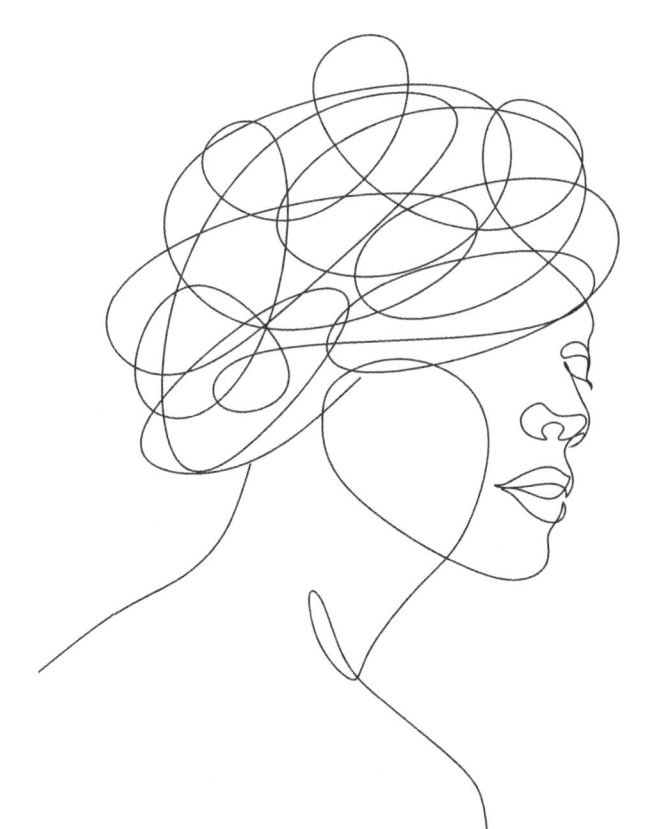

COLLABORATION: GIRLS MAY BE MORE INCLINED TO COLLABORATE WITH PEERS ON GROUP PROJECTS.

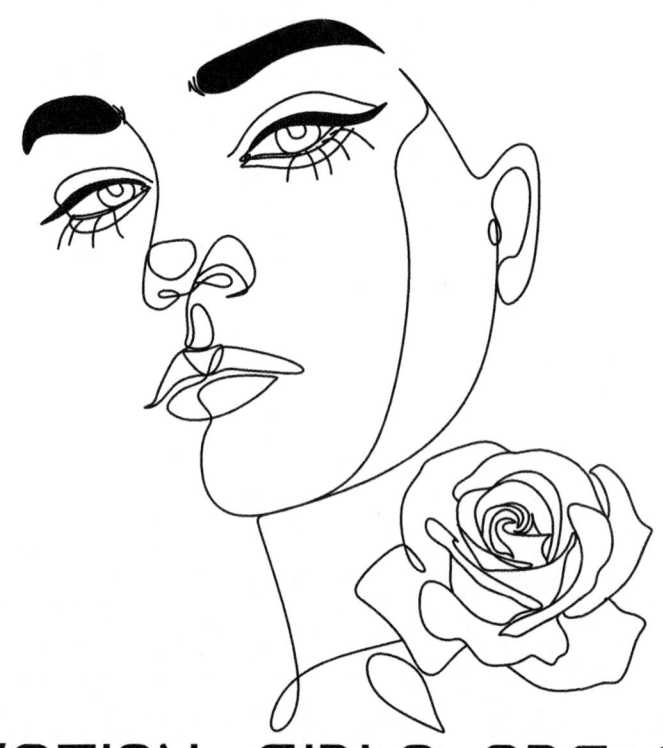

MOTIVATION: GIRLS ARE OFTEN HIGHLY MOTIVATED TO PERFORM WELL ACADEMICALLY.

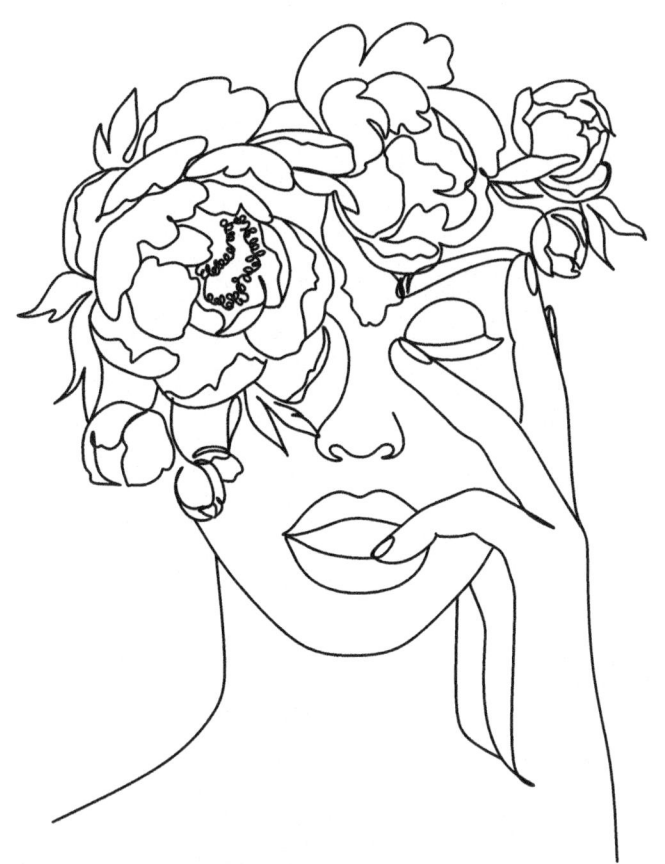

EMPATHY: A HIGHER LEVEL OF EMPATHY CAN CONTRIBUTE TO BETTER UNDERSTANDING AND PERFORMANCE IN SUBJECTS LIKE PSYCHOLOGY AND SOCIOLOGY.

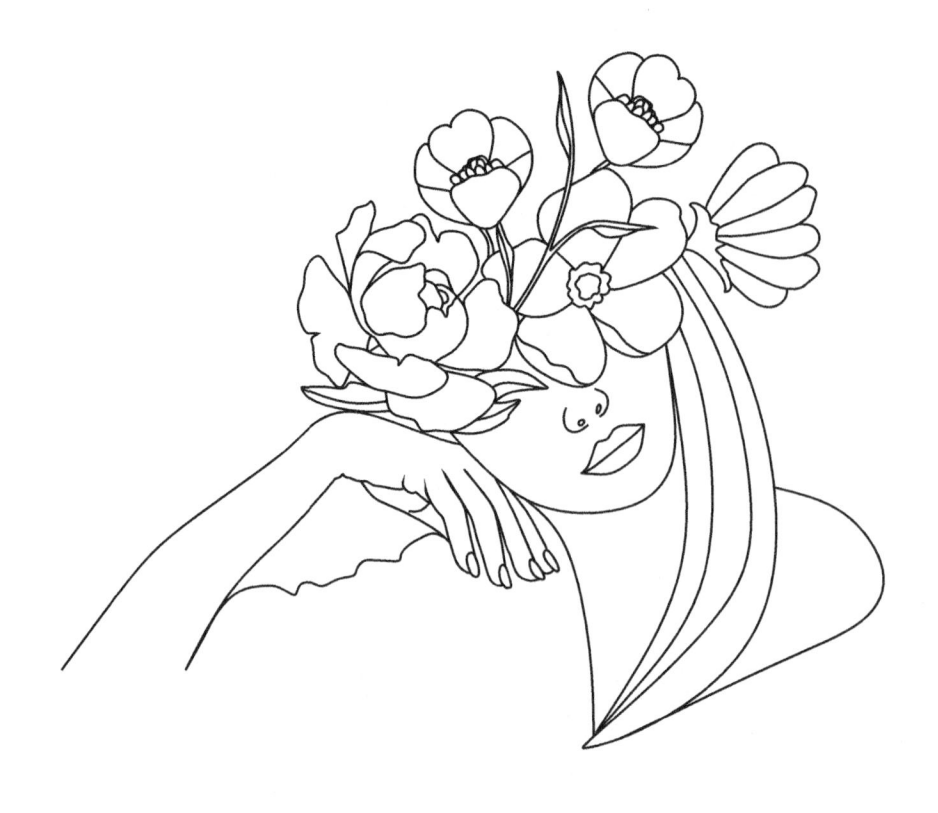

EFFECTIVE COMMUNICATION: GIRLS TEND TO EXCEL IN VERBAL COMMUNICATION SKILLS, WHICH CAN BE ADVANTAGEOUS IN LANGUAGE AND LITERATURE STUDIES.

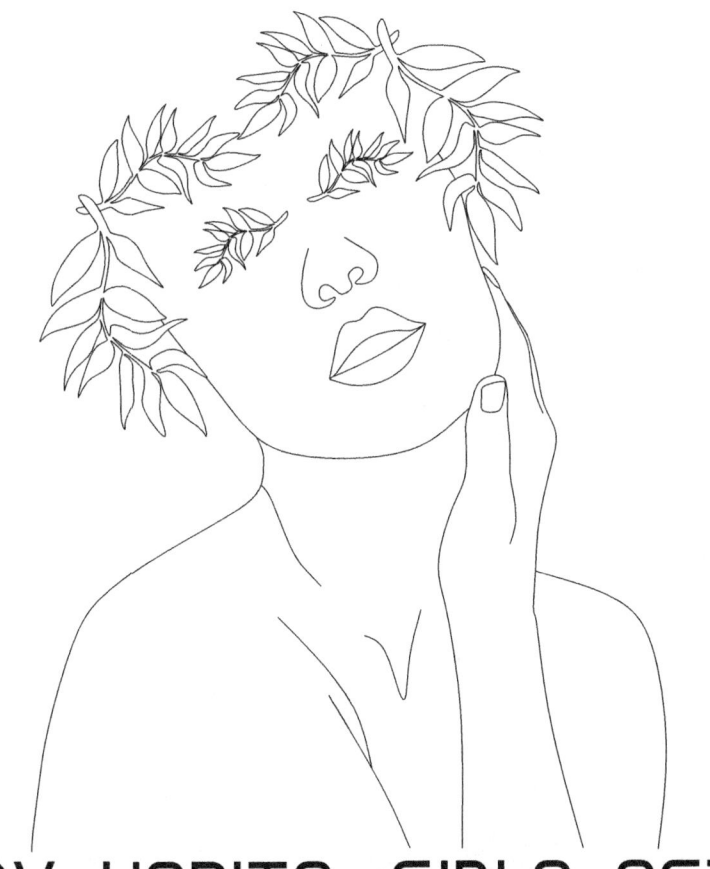

STUDY HABITS: GIRLS OFTEN
EXHIBIT STRONG STUDY HABITS,
INCLUDING BETTER TIME
MANAGEMENT AND ORGANIZATION.

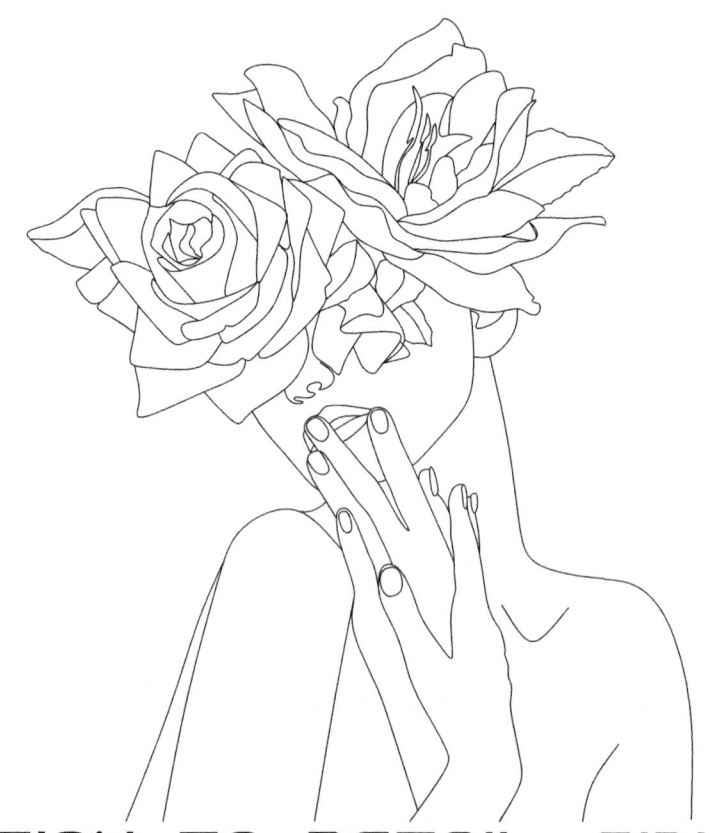

ATTENTION TO DETAIL: GIRLS MAY HAVE AN ADVANTAGE IN SUBJECTS THAT REQUIRE ATTENTION TO DETAIL AND PRECISION.

IT'S CRUCIAL TO REMEMBER THAT THESE ARE GENERAL TRENDS AND MAY NOT APPLY TO EVERY INDIVIDUAL. HEALTH IS A HIGHLY INDIVIDUALIZED EXPERIENCE, AND MANY FACTORS CONTRIBUTE TO OVERALL WELL-BEING. BOTH GENDERS HAVE UNIQUE HEALTH CHALLENGES AND STRENGTHS, AND EVERYONE SHOULD PRIORITIZE THEIR HEALTH THROUGH HEALTHY LIFESTYLE CHOICES AND REGULAR MEDICAL CHECK-UPS.

It's important to clarify that academic performance is not inherently tied to gender superiority. Both girls and boys have the potential to excel in their studies, and individual performance is influenced by various factors, including motivation, study habits, and personal interests.

INTELLIGENCE IS A COMPLEX TRAIT INFLUENCED BY VARIOUS FACTORS, AND IT IS NOT DETERMINED BY GENDER. BOTH GIRLS AND BOYS CAN EXCEL ACADEMICALLY AND INTELLECTUALLY, AND THERE IS NO EVIDENCE TO SUPPORT THE IDEA THAT ONE GENDER IS CONSISTENTLY SMARTER THAN THE OTHER.

These observations are general trends and may not apply to every individual. It's crucial to avoid making assumptions or generalizations based on gender and instead recognize the diversity of strengths and abilities in all students. Academic success is influenced by a combination of individual effort, supportive environments, and effective learning strategies.

IT IS IMPORTANT TO AVOID MAKING BROAD GENERALIZATIONS ABOUT WHAT ONE GENDER IS BETTER AT THAN THE OTHER, AS ABILITIES AND STRENGTHS VARY WIDELY AMONG INDIVIDUALS REGARDLESS OF THEIR GENDER.

Printed in Great Britain
by Amazon